Women Giving Birth

WOMEN GIVING BIRTH

PHOTOGRAPHS BY Saskia van Rees

TEXT BY Astrid Limburg and Beatrijs Smulders

WITH Dr. G.J. Kloosterman, professor of Gynecology

FOREWORD BY Suzanne Arms

CELESTIAL ARTS
Berkeley, California

Translation by Olga Smulders, copyright © 1992 by Celestial Arts Publishing
Copyedited by Cynthia Harris
Special thanks to Faye Gibson for research assistance
Suggested reading list compiled by Lynn Moen
Photographs copyright ©1984, 1992 by Saskia van Rees
Text and cover design by Nancy Austin
Layout and production by Nicole Geiger

Originally published in the Netherlands as *Baren* by Stichting Lichaamstaal

FIRST CELESTIAL ARTS PRINTING 1992

Library of Congress Cataloging-in-Publication Data

Limburg, Astrid.
    [Baren. English]
    Women giving birth / Astrid Limburg and Beatrijs Smulders;
    photographs by Saskia van Rees.
        p. cm.
    Translation of: Baren.
    Includes bibliographical references.
    ISBN 0-89087-668-1
    1. Active childbirth. 2. Active childbirth—Complications.
    3. Underwater childbirth. I. Smulders, Beatrijs. II. Rees, Saskia van. III. Title.
    RG662.L5513 1992
    618.4—dc20   91-39012
                                                                        CIP

1 2 3 4 5 6 7 8 9 10 / 96 95 94 93

CONTENTS

FOREWORD

IT WAS TEN O'CLOCK in the evening of a damp autumn day when I stepped from the taxi onto a residential street in Amsterdam with an address in my hand. It was 1974. I had flown all the way from the United States to Holland to see what was so extraordinary about the Dutch way of birth, and to document it for the book I was working on, *Immaculate Deception: A New Look at Women and Childbirth.*

I had undertaken the journey on the suggestion of two women I barely knew. One was a nurse practitioner born and raised in Holland whom I had heard speak in San Francisco at a conference on alternatives in childbirth. The feeling of ease and relaxation that she conveyed about this awesome subject went against everything I had observed and been taught as a childbirth educator in the United States.

At that time in North America, it seemed that a pregnant woman was subject to everything that could possibly make her fear her body and the process of birth—in the name of making the process modern and "safe." Birthing women were lucky if they were even fully conscious, and those who were usually witnessed the miracle of their bodies by watching it in a mirror over their heads as they lay on their backs on metal delivery tables. Gowned and masked physicians and nurses conducted the event, and fathers were routinely sent away in most hospitals. Women labored and gave birth with not one friend or family member at their sides. They were often bound to the table to keep them from touching their babies, and the babies were hustled off to spend hours or even days in the well baby nursery (an oxymoron for sure, since there is no reason that a healthy baby should be placed there). Health professionals at that time—and it is not much different today—gave lip service to birth being a normal, healthy process, but no one really believed it or acted out of that assumption.

This woman was different, however. The way in which she talked about childbirth made it sound so ordinary and natural, she got the audience to understand that there is no reason to expect a healthy woman to have problems. I was struck—more by the feeling expressed in her voice and body than by the content of her talk—that she was speaking the truth.

The other woman I spoke to was Doris Haire, who was perhaps the first lay person from the United States to critically observe the birth process in Holland. Haire had taken an early interest in childbirth practices, and wherever she and her husband traveled in the United States as a result of his work as a hospital administrator, she found a way to gain entrance into the ordinarily closed-off hospital labor and delivery units. She saw births in hospitals across North America and came to view the North American approach to birth and maternal and newborn care as "culturally warped."

When she heard I was going to take a look at birth in other cultures, Haire said, "You have to go to Holland, it is the one modernized country where I still see normal childbirth and a nearly optimal maternal-child health care system."

And so I found myself spending part of a week inside a Dutch midwifery school, the first foreign visitor ever to be invited. The school is a residential program like nursing schools were half a century ago in this country, and the students live there, eat there, and learn there. It has a clinic on campus to which pregnant and postpartum women come for care, and the babies are born in a small maternity unit that is part of the same building.

I asked to be permitted to see the entire process, beginning to end, of as many labors and births as possible, and I was awakened several times in the first two nights for the privilege. It was there that I saw medical students being taught by midwives how to conduct deliveries. I found out that they learned about the normal birth process first, before learning what can go wrong. They learned the value of supporting women and the natural process and learned to use intervention only when truly necessary.

At that time in Holland, all midwives were required as part of their training to attend home births, and many physicians in training still went out to them. I went to a home birth in a very poor section of Amsterdam and there watched a silent husband hovering awkwardly in the doorway, the midwife offering him a cup of tea to get him to stay near his partner. Every Dutch woman giving birth has the benefit of a home health visitor, a woman who comes toward the end of the birth to be an extra pair of hands and to clean up, and who then returns for the first ten days afterward to check on mother and baby (and keep records for the midwife), shop for groceries, pick up the older children from school, etc. Dutch women get paid maternity leave, and on the job, time is allowed for seeing and breastfeeding the baby in a nearby daycare center.

Through this first trip to Holland, I got a taste of what it must be like to live in a country where mothers and babies are given the care and attention they need and deserve. Everywhere I went, women talked about their childbirth experiences as being an ordinary part of life—perhaps painful and difficult at times, but quite normal and nothing to fear.

I have since been back on a number of occasions, each time seeking to discover what the pieces are that come together to make their birthing process so healthy and to see how we in North America, and in all other countries infected by the "American way of childbirth" (which views birth as a catastrophe waiting to happen), might create a better and more supportive maternity care system.

Unfortunately, those of us reared and educated and trained as health workers in North America are at a great disadvantage, as it is extremely difficult to shed cultural beliefs. Every culture has the power to warp perception of human experiences and body processes, and few cultures ever question their unique views and habits. Ours, in the United States, is no different, for all of its outward sophistication.

But it is time to question our culture as it relates to pregnancy, childbirth, and postpartum care. And it is time to change the arrogant attitude that what we do here must be best and to engineer a dramatic restructuring of our birthing system. A large and growing portion of our nation's women get inadequate health care or none at all. The cesarean surgery rate among healthy, well-educated middle-class women is well over 30 percent. More and more obstetricians are leaving obstetrics, yet major medical associations are trying to restrict or eliminate the practice of midwifery and other allied health professions.

I was fortunate to see both the birthing process in Holland and home births in the United States, for I discovered that birth was possible with no intervention, no wearing of a hospital gown, no pubic shave or enema (both still routine in the 1970s), no IV drip, no drugs, no episiotomy. In so many of the American births I have seen, the women labored and labored, with slow progress, and pushed and pushed and pushed for hours. Dutch women do not seem to have the difficulty American women do and have fewer complications with their pregnancies.

Women Giving Birth helps to explain why. It is a celebration of the Dutch way of birth and its impact upon ordinary people: women, men, babies, siblings, and entire families. The stories in it—by the people themselves—are candid and revealing and very relevant. *Women Giving Birth* is a window onto a whole different way of looking at birth—as the healthy and normal process that we hear about but see so little of. It is extremely valuable for anyone considering having a baby or who is preparing for childbirth.

—SUZANNE ARMS

Women Giving Birth

Delivering with Both Feet on the Ground

IN SEVERAL AREAS OF HOLLAND, midwives and the women under their care began to experiment with a number of spontaneous delivery positions used prior to the eighteenth century that had been almost forgotten by Western medicine. During the past two decades, these midwives have gained invaluable experience with vertical birth, the most natural and ancient method of delivery. (Third World nations have continued to use vertical positions for childbearing.) Exploration for alternatives to the current conventional birthing position did not come out of the blue; the disadvantages of delivering while lying on one's back, in the supine position, have long been known.

First, a lot of time and energy is wasted on an unnecessary battle against gravity. Lying on her back—legs in the air, knees pulled up toward the chest and spread apart, chin on chest—is extremely tiring for a woman in labor. In essence, this is a horizontal squatting position, which does open up the pelvis and relax the muscles of the pelvic floor, though not as much as squatting when one is vertical (*see* Increased Mobility of the Pelvis, page 5). But "squatting" while on one's back turns gravity into a hindrance rather than using it to assist delivery. The infeasibility of giving birth in the supine position is made very clear when one considers the position assumed for defecating, another expulsive function of the body. We sit upright on the toilet, and when no facilities are available—on a camping trip, for example—we squat. It never occurs to us to lie down to have a bowel movement, and if someone suggested that we should do so, we wouldn't take them seriously. If it weren't for cultural conditioning, the idea of delivering supine—and thereby hampering a physiological process by going against the law of gravity—would strike us as equally absurd.

Pressure placed on main blood vessels within the pelvic cavity is another major disadvantage of supine delivery. The baby's weight as well as that of the amniotic fluid and placenta presses onto the vessels that provide the blood flow into the placenta, blood flow which is vital for the child's oxygenation.

In the seventies, many midwives rejected the supine position and switched to the semisitting position in which the woman half sits and half lies, supported by pillows, with her legs slightly bent and her feet flat on the mattress. A new problem arose; in this position, the woman's weight tends to restrict the birth opening, leaving too little room for the baby's head and shoulders. If a woman were to remain in this position, she would experience an uncomfortable counterpressure from the mattress as the head descended and the anus began to bulge. This position is particularly unsuitable for a first-time mother, who must exert more strength to push her baby through the unprepared birth canal. If she is halfway between sitting and lying down, she cannot brace herself sufficiently. It is not without reason, after pushing in this position for a while without success, she is advised to lie down farther to provide more room for the head to pass through.

Midwives are finding that an increasing number of women prefer to remain positioned vertically during delivery. Squatting, sitting, kneeling, and standing facilitate the birth process for both mother and child. Awareness of the advantages of vertical birth is growing among doctors. In some hospitals, vertical delivery is already customary.

It goes without saying that a birthing position can be effective only if it is simple to assume, easily maintained, and very stable. During deliveries attended by midwives, many women intuitively went into the supported squat. The supported squatting position, because of its simplicity and stability, is an obvious position to choose. A partner sits on a sofa, chair, or bed behind the woman, who squats between her partner's legs. She rests her arms on their thighs. If the pushing is prolonged for any reason, as it often is with a first child, the woman is supported by a small birthchair or by a bucket with a wide edge on which she can sit comfortably. This extra support is usually removed the moment the head presents itself, because during vertical deliveries from that point on, many women no longer need to push.

Some women shy away from the squatting position because they've heard the misconception that Western women have become totally unaccustomed to squatting and that they should take special courses to learn to squat from the third month of pregnancy on. Most women who have delivered in a squatting position have, in fact, practiced very little. Exercise during pregnancy is helpful but is not necessary.

A delivery in the supported squatting position is a joint effort in which both the woman and her partner are actively involved. Besides providing physical support during the squatting, the partner can instill in the woman a sense of security when she leans back to rest between contractions. Together they watch the child being born.

More and more often a woman will invite a girlfriend or someone with whom the couple is very close to attend the delivery. Their presence adds an extra dimension to the birth. Childbirth becomes more of a communal event. Having a girlfriend present gives the woman who is delivering a feeling of security, which helps relax her body, and the woman attending has a wonderful opportunity to experience a birth first-hand, gaining direct transference of knowledge rather than having to extract all her information from books.

The current developments in vertical birth have taken place primarily in women's homes. This is understandable; for at home, in her own environment, surrounded by people of her choice, a woman feels free to take on her own position and to follow the signals of her body. Not only is the position altered but the whole atmosphere around the birth changes. Consequently, the idea to which we have been conditioned for two centuries, that a bed is necessary for birthing, is no longer accepted as true. Hospital delivery rooms in which vertical deliveries are standard practice contain no beds. Bedrooms, often small and the chilliest rooms of the house, are usually less than ideal locations for home deliveries. A woman should choose the spot in her home that is most comfortable and warm.

The differences in emotions between a woman in a horizontal position and a woman in a vertical position are profound. In the vertical position, she has "both feet on the ground": she knows exactly what is happening, remains more herself, and is more involved with the delivery. The upright position is an optimistic position, making her feel strong. She can trust her body, which has been made to give birth, and deliver with her own strength. She has equal status with those around her. This is not the case when a women is in the supine position. She lies in a bed as if ill, and people tower above her, making her feel small and dependent. When the delivery does not go smoothly, she tends to surrender to the specialist and gives up responsibility.

Quite an unexpected development in terms of the mother's first contact with the newborn child was made possible by the vertical delivery: she can see her child immediately and is the first person to hold her baby. When a woman delivers in the supine position, the midwife must actively assist the baby's birth. It has been our experience that such intervention is usually unnecessary with vertical deliveries. The child is born by itself, due to the contractions and gravity, and the midwife merely catches it. The baby slides onto an obstetric pad on the floor in front of the mother. There are no time pressures; a woman can adhere to her own rhythm, recovering her breath and becoming attuned to her child at her own pace.

MAKING ARRANGEMENTS FOR THE DELIVERY

Early in your pregnancy, it is wise to discuss the type of delivery you envision with your midwife or obstetrician and to come to full agreement with her or him. To find out during the delivery that your opinions about giving birth don't correspond with their routine would be an unpleasant surprise. If you feel the midwife or doctor should stay in the background and leave you to initiate events, you should talk about this. Both parties must be absolutely clear and straightforward to ensure that the experience of birth is fulfilling to you and the others involved. Above all, keep in mind that this is your delivery, your child.

THE FOLLOWING ARE some of the issues you will want to raise:

WHO WILL BE at the delivery?

Do you want only your partner to be present, or do you want to invite a friend, sister, mother, or other relative.

If you have other children, do you feel they should be there, or would their presence distract or inhibit you?

WHERE ARE YOU going to deliver?

At home or in a hospital? If in a hospital, visit several in advance and ask about their regulations. Choose the one with which you feel most comfortable.

If you decide to deliver at home, in what room will you give birth: the living room, the bedroom, the bathroom? Remember to take into consideration the size of the room, the noise level, and the heating. You will also want to decide if taking a bath or shower during labor or delivery sounds appealing to you.

WHICH POSITIONS appeal to you?

Will you squat, stand, or kneel? One of the misconceptions about squatting is that one must practice from the third month of pregnancy. Although useful, exercise is not necessary. Most women interviewed in this book who delivered vertically did not do squatting exercises.

WHAT DO YOU WANT to happen during your first contact with your child?

Do you want anybody else to touch the baby besides you and your partner?

Do you want to bathe the baby yourself or would you like your partner to do this? Would you like to get into the tub with the baby?

PART I

Vertical Delivery

History

THROUGHOUT THE world until the eighteenth century, the vertical delivery was the most prevalent way to give birth. The illustrations that follow are representations of women from different cultures and periods of history during delivery. Invariably, the woman in labor is depicted in a vertical position, either squatting, sitting, or standing.

Ancient Egypt provides numerous representations of birth. The woman usually sat on a primitive birthchair, made of bricks, or kneeled. A drawing after a bas-relief on the temple of Esneh (Figure 1) shows Cleopatra giving birth on her knees.

We come upon similar kneeling positions in Greco-Roman mythology. Figure 2 portrays Leto's childbirth. In order to

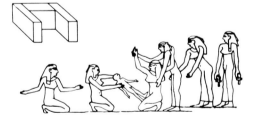

Figure 1

deliver, Leto had to flee to the island of Delos because she was chased by the jealous Hera. (Leto was expecting a baby by Zeus, Hera's spouse and the supreme Greek deity.) Leto could be delivered only with the help of the birth goddess Eileithyia. Leto is often depicted giving birth in a kneeling position. After nine long days

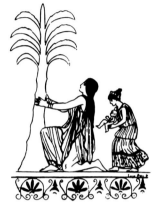

Figure 2

of labor with "one knee resting on the soft grass," she gave birth to twins, Artemis and Apollo.

Representations of vertical deliveries from the Middle Ages show that a low

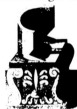

Figure 3

birthchair was used. The midwife sat in front of the woman on a small stool. Helpers, on either side or behind, supported the woman giving birth. Birthchairs ranged from handsomely decorated pieces such as Figure 3 (Moinet, Paul. "L'énigme de la Papesse Jeanne." *Æsculape* [January 1929]: 320.) to simple wooden chairs that were owned by the community and lent out for deliveries. Figure 4 shows a Renaissance delivery on such a birthchair.

The woman in labor sits bolt upright,

supported from behind by another woman, while the midwife, as was customary in those days, sits in front of her and with hands under the woman's skirts "blindly" performs the delivery. (Roslin, Eucharius. *Der swangern Frauwen und Hebammen Rosegarten* [The Pregnant Women's and Midwife's Rosegarden]. 1513.) Sometimes the birthchair was replaced by the "living birthchair," and the laboring woman would sit on the midwife's lap for a "lap delivery."

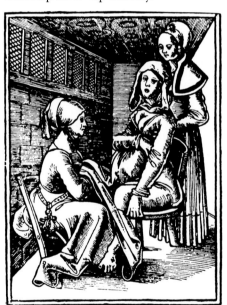

Figure 4

Figure 5 shows a Sioux delivery. The woman, supported by her partner, stands to deliver, and the midwife sits behind her to catch the child. (Witkowski, G. *Histoire des Accouchements de Tout Les Peuples* [World History of Giving Birth], Paris, 1887.)

An abundance of birth scenes showing deliveries in a variety of vertical po-

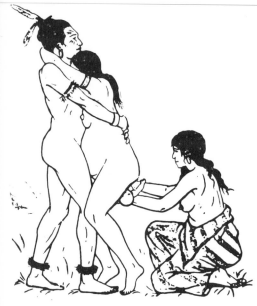

Figure 5

sitions comes from Robert Felkin's late nineteenth century report, "Notes on Labour in Central Africa." In Figure 6, a woman in labor sits on a tree trunk by the riverside. Bystanders make music to avert evil spirits. Figure 7 shows a delivery in a sitting position; a helper exerts considerable pressure on the woman's body from behind. Figures 8 and 9 prove that standing during delivery was practiced in Africa as well. (Felkin, Robert W. "Notes on

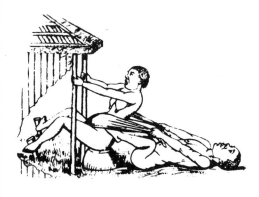

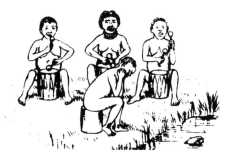

Figure 6 & 7

Labour in Central Africa." *Edinburgh Medical Journal* [April 1884].)

FROM VERTICAL TO HORIZONTAL

In the seventeenth and eighteenth centuries, opinions about how to deliver began to diverge from the spontaneous vertical positions that had always been used. Europe flourished economically, and the increased wealth gave a boost to education and science. Until that time, deliveries had been solely the realm of women, and experience was the main source of knowledge. Science's first step into the domain of obstetrics was the publication of *Traite des Maladies des Femmes Grosses et de celles qui sont nouvellement ac-*

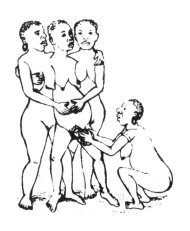

Figure 8

couchees [Treatise on the Diseases Affecting Women During and Post Partum] in 1668 by the French obstetrician François Mauriceau in which the anatomy and physiology of female reproductive organs were described in detail. Solutions were sought to help women through difficult labors and to reduce maternal and infant death rates. At the end of the seventeenth century, Mauriceau introduced the obstetric bed that eventually replaced the traditional birthchair. Evidently, interventions such as internal and external rotation of the baby, removal of a dead fetus, and, later, the application of forceps could be done most effectively when a woman was lying on her back. Naturally, these measures were applied only in problematic deliveries.

Over time, however, even uncomplicated deliveries took place in a supine position. The fetal stethoscope, used to listen to fetal heart tones, was invented around 1850. With this instrument, the baby's heart tones can be heard best when the mother is lying on her back because there is less movement. More and more often, even during normal deliveries, the emphasis was placed on monitoring the unborn in order to intervene if necessary. Fetal heart tones were checked frequently during the delivery, making it essential for the woman to be supine. In this way, with an advance in technology, albeit an invention of incalculable value, even women whose labors progressed without problems were delivered in a horizontal position.

The invention of the fetal stethoscope explains the change from the vertical to the supine position for deliveries without complications much more plausibly than other theories concerning this obstetric development, such as the tale of the sexually perverse Louis XIV or the explanation that women have been "put on their backs" since the arrival of men in obstetrics merely to facilitate the obstetrician's job. The story about Louis XIV claims that he derived sexual gratification by watching from behind a curtain as his mistresses gave birth. If these women had delivered fully dressed on a birthchair, he would have seen very little. To ensure that the king would have more opportunity to observe,

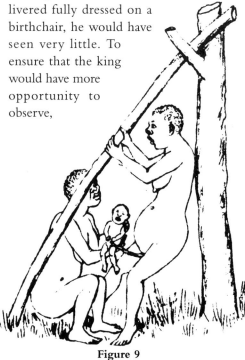

Figure 9

the court physician supposedly convinced these women that childbirth would be easier if they laid on a table.

Although we don't accept the obstetrician's desire for convenience or to dominate the delivering woman as the reason behind the switch to the supine position, we do believe this position tended to appeal to the sense of authority of those assisting the woman in labor, increasing the chance that the birth process was orchestrated to suit them. Within this framework, the woman does not give birth—the doctor delivers her of her child and preferably of her pain as well. The supine position exaggerated the vulnerability of the woman giving birth and paved the way for interventionary care. In the United States, beginning in the mid-nineteenth century, this attitude resulted in the practice of putting women whose conditions indicated they would have routine deliveries under general anesthesia. Due to improved health conditions of women and developments of medical science, maternal and infant mortality rates dropped drastically. Doctors' successes at applying new medical techniques increased faith in medical intervention and augmented the authority of obstetricians and their medical staffs. Unfortunately, the advantages of natural delivery in a vertical position for women who didn't require intervention, the majority, fell into oblivion.

At the end of the 1960s, the Doppler apparatus was invented. This instrument sends out ultrasonic signals (high-frequency waves that the human ear cannot hear) of the unborn child's heart and converts them into sound so the fetal heart tones can be heard. With this technology, the fetal heart tones can be monitored during or between contractions while the woman is in any position. Since the Doppler apparatus has replaced the fetal stethoscope, no convincing argument remains for a normal birth to take place in a horizontal position.

Naturally, transitions in standard obstetric practice cannot be expected to occur overnight. Medical information and technology alone do not destroy a deep-rooted practice of several centuries. It will take time for society as well as for those who work in the field to let go of horizontal or semi-horizontal delivery procedures and to begin thinking and working differently. But over the past decade, more and more prospective parents with the full support of their midwives or obstetricians have chosen to deliver vertically, a positive indication of our readiness to return to this traditional, logical position for giving birth.

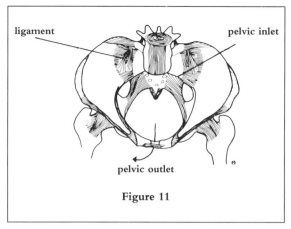

Figure 11

Advantages of Vertical Delivery

PHYSIOLOGICAL ADVANTAGES

Increased Mobility of the Pelvis

The pelvis, the base of the trunk, consists of four bones that are linked by six ligaments, or bands of strong connective tissue. This bony circle rests on the thigh bones.

In obstetrics, we speak of the pelvis

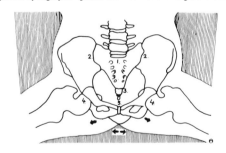

1. joint between the lower back and sacrum
2. sacroiliac joint (joint between the sacrum and ilium)
3. joint between the sacrum and coccyx
4. hip joint
5. pubic symphysis (joint between the two pubic bones)

Figure 10*

as consisting of (from top to bottom) the upper pelvis (pelvic brim), pelvic inlet, and the pelvic outlet. The child's head rests in the upper pelvis throughout gestation. At the end of pregnancy, his or her head works its way down through the

* This figure and those that follow are from the perspective of looking down through the pelvis from above.

pelvic inlet, and the baby arrives in this world through the pelvic outlet.

Due to hormonal changes toward the end of pregnancy, the connective tissue of tendons and ligaments in and around the bones of the pelvis relaxes, and the pelvis, normally a rigid tube, becomes a dynamic and flexible structure (Figure 11).

During delivery, a woman can influence the degree of the pelvis's mobility by changing her position. Squatting, bending at the knees and spreading the legs out far enough from the hips—about eight inches on each side, a distance that comes naturally to a pregnant woman in order to maintain her balance—puts traction on the otherwise relaxed pubic symphysis and increases the pubic arch, or space under the pubic bones. Because of this flexibility, the pelvic brim adjusts to the baby's head, which brings about an early turning of the head and promotes rotation in the birth canal.

In addition, the sacroiliac joint gives the sacrum, the bone forming the back wall of the pelvis, certain flexibility. When the trunk bends forward, as it does in the squatting position, the sacrum turns on its axis and opens up the pelvis from behind, increasing the width of the pelvic outlet.

Figure 12 illustrates that as the upper part of the sacrum, which is connected to the lower back, moves forward, the lower sacrum is stretched back unless a person

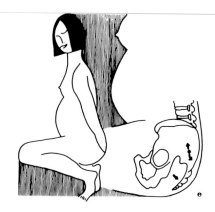

Figure 12

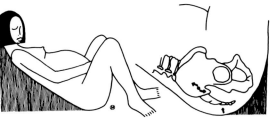

Figure 13

sits on a hard surface, in which case it is pushed forward toward the center of the birth canal. The coccyx, or tailbone, located at the lower end of the sacrum, responds in like by either moving back out of the way or pressing forward.

In the semisitting position shown in Figure 13, pressure is exerted in a way that flattens the pelvis. To exert strength in this position, a woman uses the coccyx as a push-off point; thus, the tailbone is not able to move out of the way because of the counterpressure produced by the bed. In turn, this pressure is transmitted to both parts of the pubic arch, pushing the pubic bones toward each other. Furthermore, when sitting like this, a woman's thighs usually are not spread apart far enough to put tension on the

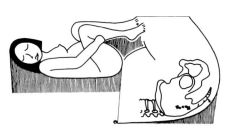

Figure 14

pubic symphysis. The result: the pubic arch is not stretched at all.

The supine position (Figure 14) is a better position for delivery than the semisitting position because the back rather than the coccyx is used as the push-off point. When a woman lies down and pulls her knees toward her chest, the coccyx is unobstructed and the upper part of the body is bent in a way that increases the size of the pelvic opening. The major drawback of the supine delivery is that gravity is not used to the woman's advantage.

Working with Gravity

During a delivery, several forces bring about the birth of a child: uterine contractions, the breath in conjunction with the abdominal muscles, the dynamics of the pelvis, and gravity. Self-confidence enables the woman to surrender to what is happening within her body and to rally these sources of strength. In the

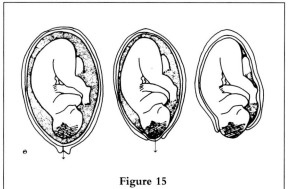

Figure 15

horizontal delivery, gravity works against the other forces, but in a vertical delivery, it works in conjunction with the rest of the birth process and promotes the child's birth.

DURING CERVICAL DILATATION: A contraction moves like a wave through the womb: it increases in strength, reaches a peak, and diminishes gradually. While the cervix is closed, the force of contractions is distributed equally over the entire womb. During the first stage of labor, cervical dilatation, contractions cause the effaced cervix (*see* page 9) to open slowly,

dilatating slightly more with each contraction as in Figure 15.

Over the course of cervical dilatation, contractions lengthen and increase in intensity and frequency. The womb becomes narrower during a contraction, which raises the intrauterine pressure. The

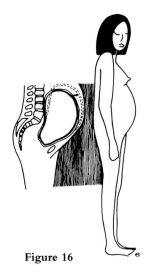

Figure 16

baby's heart reacts to this pressure change. Then the contraction subsides and is followed by a break. The interval between contractions is vital because the pressure on the baby and the placenta is relieved temporarily. Of particular importance is the recovery of the blood flow through the placenta, which is at its lowest level at the peak of a contraction.

The shape and position of the uterus during a contraction—extended, lifted, and forward—transforms the womb into a continuation of the pelvic axis so the baby's head pushes against the cervix effectively. When a woman is in the vertical position as shown in Figure 16, gravity does not counteract the forward movement of the uterus during a contraction.

In the semisitting or the supine position, the uterine muscles must exert

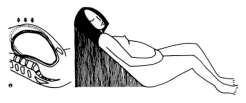

Figure 17

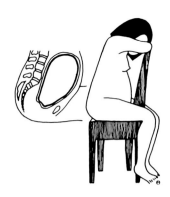

Figure 18

themselves to the utmost during each contraction to lift the womb against the force of gravity (Figure 17). This takes energy away from cervical dilatation, which will last longer than necessary and fatigue both mother and child needlessly.

Figure 18 illustrates that when a woman leans forward as she sits, the womb is already tilted slightly so no energy needs to be diverted from the contraction to move the uterus to this position. In this manner, gravity increases the effectiveness of the contractions and accelerates cervical dilatation.

DURING THE PUSHING STAGE: The supported squatting position is sometimes considered to be too fatiguing, if not im-

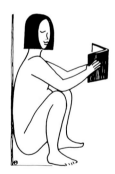

Figure 19

possible, for Western women during the pushing stage. In our culture, we sit on chairs and are not used to prolonged squatting. People in other cultures squat when at rest as well as when working. During pregnancy, it is advisable to become comfortable with the position. Squatting—flat footed with back against a wall (Figure 19), starting with one to two minutes at a time and building up to

ten to fifteen minutes—each day is a useful exercise.

In the vertical position, the transition from dilatation contractions to the actual pushing runs a more natural course. During maximum dilatation, the baby's head pushes with greater force because of gravity, so the woman really feels the urge to push. Teaching the "pushing technique" usually becomes superfluous since women in this position almost always start to push intuitively during the peak of a contraction. There is absolutely no need to tell a woman who is in a vertical position to "take a deep breath, close off throat, put

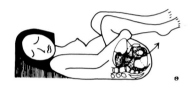

Figure 20

chin on chest," preferably three times during a contraction. Unless coached to push differently, the tendency of a woman delivering supine is to substitute making noises from the throat for using the abdominal muscles to move the baby. Pushing from the abdomen in a vertical position is more effective for two reasons: firstly, the abdominal muscles need not work against gravity, and secondly, the woman does not need to lift up her head. This means intra-abdominal and intra-thoracic pressure, pressure between the mother's neck and abdomen, will not rise as much when she is vertical so there is less chance of hindering her circulation

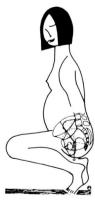

Figure 21

or that of her baby. (*See* Circulation of Mother and Child, belows.)

In the supine position, the final portion of the birth canal bends upward as shown in Figure 20. Because the woman pushes against gravity when she lies down, the pelvic floor and perineum, the area between anus and vagina, become a "mountain" over which she must push the baby.

Figure 21 illustrates that pushing with gravity is the line of least resistance.

CIRCULATION OF MOTHER AND CHILD: Nearly all expectant women from about six months of pregnancy on have experienced feeling lightheaded, short of breath, and anxious after lying on their backs for as short a period of time as five minutes to half an hour. In the supine position, the heavy womb rests on the inferior vena cava, a large vein that returns blood to the heart, causing a severe drop of venous blood to the heart and a decrease of oxygenated blood to the aorta. Ultimately, arterial blood pressure decreases and the woman feels faint, but these symptoms disappear when she turns onto her side. The hypotension also affects the blood flow through the placenta, which means the child's oxygen supply is insufficient when the mother is supine.

As mentioned previously, the increase of intrauterine pressure at the peak of a contraction reduces placental blood flow to its lowest level. The blood flow improves between contractions, and the child can "recover its breath" when a woman is upright. Delivering in a vertical position prevents circulation problems for both mother and child. In the supine position, however, the relaxed uterus falls onto the inferior vena cava during this recovery stage. A fetus in prime condition can bear quite a bit, and, in general, the supine delivery does not lead to infants born in noticeably poor condition. Nevertheless, it is not inconceivable that the child may suffer unnecessarily during an extended supine delivery.

The vertical position is the optimal delivery position not only because it co-operates with a woman's physiology and gravity but, in great part, because of the positive influence it has on her emotional sense of well-being. When a woman squats to deliver, she is at eye level with those attending her. Between contractions she is their social equal. She remains in contact with what is happening around her and can indicate her desires, can consult others, or can wait quietly for the next contraction.

Another psychological benefit of delivering upright is that she is familiar with pushing from this position as she assumes it daily to defecate. Pushing while supine is unfamiliar; in addition, when on her back, the woman lies with her legs spread apart, her vagina uncovered and exposed. During the pushing, feces generally leave the body, and, not surprisingly, most women are humiliated to have bystanders, especially strangers, present during this intimate act. She may experience feelings

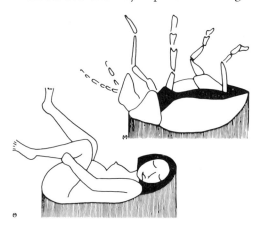

of shame and loneliness, and the attempt to suppress these emotions can disturb her self-confidence. By squatting and bending slightly forward, she does not feel as vulnerable because she is less exposed.

Giving birth in the supine position often makes women feel passive and helpless, a sensation sometimes compared with the helplessness of a beetle on its back. An inherent danger of the supine position is that a woman is reduced to the "object" from which a child is delivered. The helpers turn into spectators around a vagina, which is suddenly pronounced to be public territory. Assistants may not see the whole woman—a physical and emotional being—when she is supine.

In a vertical delivery, the woman giving birth directs the process and is active physically and mentally. "Bystanders" become partners who assist her in her efforts. Since a woman understands intuitively how she should push from this position, she is much less dependent on instructions from others. This boosts her self-confidence and enables her to deliver her child with her own strength.

Vertical Delivery in Practice

Delivering Better: The Dutch System

Historically, the Dutch have preferred natural birth, and midwives and obstetricians have gone to the woman's home for the delivery. A principal component of obstetric care is the maternity nurse, who cares for mother and child in their home for ten days after delivery. In most of the rest of the Western world, women are discouraged from delivering at home. In some states in the United States, giving birth at home is even illegal.

The Dutch tradition of home delivery is made possible by a unique and extensive prenatal care system for all women. This system protects the healthy woman from unnecessary medical intervention. Midwives screen women carefully during pregnancy, and those women who risk having complications (approximately 30 percent) are referred to an obstetrician and must deliver in a well-equipped hospital. All other women, the majority, have the choice of delivering at home or in a hospital.

Since most disorders can be diagnosed during prenatal care, and hospital deliveries planned in advance for women whose situations make them more likely to need intervention, the success of home deliveries can be predicted with a high degree of certainty. Nonetheless, something un-expected may happen during the delivery that requires a woman to be transported to a hospital. Labor is interrupted by the trip, and the woman may feel tired from the contractions and disappointed that the delivery is not going as planned. A woman needs to gather her strength at such a moment. The end is in sight, and there is comfort in knowing that a portion of the delivery took place in her own environment. Her contentment with the delivery should not depend upon whether the birth followed a natural course, but rather upon the knowledge that she did everything within her power to bring the delivery to a happy and safe end, wherever and however it took place. In addition, the tradition of home delivery has had a positive influence on hospital obstetric care. In hospitals in Holland, unlike countries where routine deliveries take place in hospitals, a woman's individuality is respected.

To Be Pregnant Is to Be a Little Bit Healthier

The saying "pregnancy is a healthy disease" gives the false impression that a pregnant woman is ill, when, in fact, she is slightly more healthy than a nonpregnant woman. During pregnancy, the body functions optimally, but being pregnant takes extra energy, energy the child uses to develop and grow. A woman's body makes her aware of this early in the pregnancy. Fatigue is one of the most common complaints among expectant women.

As long as she listens to the signals from her body, a woman can continue to have an active life during pregnancy. She should treat herself to extra rest and to nutritious meals. If she does not, she will not feel well. In addition to having a healthy lifestyle, being well informed about what happens during pregnancy, and especially during labor and delivery, is important. Ignorance promotes fear, tension, and insecurity, which undermine a woman's self-confidence when she gives birth. To boost their confidence, women can read books on childbearing and attend pregnancy courses where they will come into contact with other pregnant women. Exchanging experiences and information gives a woman reassurance. She should search for a class that helps her ready herself for the type of delivery she desires. In these courses, she will have the opportunity to become familiar with squatting, breathing, and relaxation techniques; however, a woman should never feel that she cannot deliver without first "being trained."

PRECONTRACTIONS

The cervix is formed of strong, tough tissue, comparable to the tissue at the tip of the nose. This tissue keeps the womb closed tightly during gestation so its contents will not be expelled prematurely. Due to hormonal changes and to precontractions, the spout-shaped cervix softens and becomes supple, allowing it to change shape slowly. This process, called effacement, often begins during the final weeks of pregnancy and prepares the cervix for dilatation.

Precontractions are minor, irregular contractions of the uterus. Sometimes precontractions are called "false labor," a term that can be discouraging for women and is also misleading since they do have some effect on effacement. Ordinarily, precontractions can be distinguished easily from Braxton-Hicks contractions, or the so-called hard stomach, which are painless and strengthen the uterine muscle for delivery.

Women pregnant for the first time often find it hard to distinguish between precontractions and contractions of cervical dilatation. A precontraction lasts about thirty seconds, and successive contractions do not increase in intensity; whereas contractions of cervical dilatation increase in length, until at the end of dilatation they last a minute to a minute and a half, and as the dilatation progresses, the contractions become stronger and succeed one another more rapidly.

It is important for a woman to be aware of the differences between precontractions and contractions of cervical dilatation. Precontractions do not always announce the beginning of delivery; they do not cause cervical dilatation but may, in the course of time, usher in dilatation contractions, or may subside, disappearing entirely, and the delivery may not occur for another week or so.

HOW DOES LABOR ANNOUNCE ITSELF?

Within the uterus, the child lives in a kind of balloon called the amniotic membranes. These two translucent elastic membranes hold about a liter of amniotic fluid at the end of pregnancy. The fluid and membranes form a buffer for the fetus. During pregnancy, the cervix is closed off by a tough plug of mucous; this mucous plug and the amniotic membranes protect the fetus against infection from the outside world. The mucous plug becomes liquidy at the end of pregnancy. As effacement occurs, the plug leaves the body along with a small amount of blood. This occurrence is called the "show." The discharge, which in most women leaves the vagina a drop at a time, amounts to so little that it can sometimes go unnoticed. Although in most cases labor starts with dilatation contractions or with a show, approximately 10 percent of the time it begins with the rupture of the amniotic membranes, or the waters breaking, which usually happens at night. Occasionally, the amniotic membranes do not rupture on their own and must be broken by the midwife or obstetrician because they would otherwise protrude into the vagina during the pushing.

Near the end of pregnancy, it is important for the midwife to monitor the position of the child's head. If the head is high in the pelvis when labor begins, there is a possibility of umbilical cord prolapse, or the cord lying low in the pelvis. In this position, the cord—the child's source of oxygen—may be compressed or blocked completely as the contractions force the head downward. If at the woman's previous checkup the head had not yet descended properly into the pelvic brim, she should call her midwife immediately the moment her waters break. The midwife will examine her to see if the umbilical cord prolapsed when the amniotic fluid left the vagina. A prolapsed cord is a dangerous situation and, fortunately, does not occur often. Another reason for a woman to call her midwife immediately is if the amniotic fluid is green or brown rather than clear. This means the child has been or still is short of oxygen, causing him or her to defecate into the fluid. The midwife will come right away to check the baby's heart tones.

When a woman's waters break and the amniotic fluid is clear and the head has descended properly, she should glance at the clock and note the time the membranes ruptured, then try to go back to sleep. She can wait until morning to tell the midwife what happened during the night.

Once the membranes have ruptured, the uterine environment is open to the outside and infection is possible. Good hygiene is necessary. The woman should refrain from taking a bath until cervical dilatation is in progress, although a shower at this point is fine, and she should put nothing into her vagina. Generally, the child will be born within twenty-four hours of the waters breaking. If not, the woman may need to be admitted to a hospital because the chance of infection increases. At the hospital, contraction-stimulating hormones will be administered to speed up the delivery.

CERVICAL DILATATION

When giving birth, a woman literally and figuratively "opens up." During cervical dilatation, the hormone oxytocin is secreted, which causes the uterus to contract powerfully. Changes over which a woman has no control take place within her body. We are accustomed to managing many aspects of our lives, so surrendering to the birth process can be difficult. A woman must remember that her body is designed for childbirth and can handle the pain that goes along with it. When she fights the pain, her mind blocks the body's coping mechanisms. Once a woman stops resisting the physical sensations, she enters slowly into a state of mind that allows her instincts to take over. The key is to accept the pain as it comes and to trust that it will dissipate. However contradictory it may sound, welcoming discomfort rather than cursing it gives a woman the self-confidence and strength to go on. In addition, when she is not tense, her body produces morphinelike hormones called endorphins. This natural painkiller alters a woman's consciousness during labor and delivery, letting her be open to this new experience.

In order to relax during the birth process, which enables her body to produce oxytocin and endorphins, a woman needs warmth, the comfort of familiar faces surrounding her, and freedom to move. As soon as the contractions have begun, she should make sure she is warm. There is some truth in the Dutch saying, "A cold woman does not deliver." Turning up the heat and putting on a sweater and thick socks will help speed up her progress. Doing light chores around the house during early dilatation, when the contractions are relatively weak, distracts her so she won't stare at the clock as she waits for her next contraction. She should allow herself time to get used to the contractions before calling the friends and family she has asked to attend the delivery. Some women may want to call the midwife or doctor immediately upon the onset of contractions, while others choose to wait awhile. Most likely, the midwife will perform a vaginal examination when she arrives. She will feel how soft the cervix has become, to what extent the cervix has opened, and how far the baby's head has descended. This procedure can be done easily when the woman sits on a birthchair, and in this position, the examination is less uncomfortable because the perineum is relaxed and the vagina is more open. After several hours of contractions, a woman may be burning with curiosity to know how far dilatation has progressed; the midwife may be equally curious but reluctant to check vaginally until she feels it is necessary because each examination increases the chance of infection.

During the contractions and the actual delivery, choosing a position that is totally satisfying at the moment—whether it be squatting, kneeling, standing, walking, or lying down—is of utmost importance. During cervical dilatation, we encourage women to remain positioned vertically. If a woman lies down during contractions, she will not feel inclined to change her position because she is stiff, and she must be persuaded to get into a vertical position at the beginning of pushing. Once she squats, however, she will be struck by the simple logic and comfort of this position. *How comfortable* and *What a relief* is what we often hear.

A woman must keep in mind that she is giving birth to her baby with her own strength, and the people around her are there to assist; the midwife and others are

When to Call the Midwife or Obstetrician

EVERY WOMAN REACTS to the onset of dilatation contractions in her own way. Some women prefer to hold off notifying the midwife or doctor and to share early contractions with only a partner. Others feel more secure if they call for medical advice right away.

A woman should call for assistance immediately in the following circumstances:
• her amniotic fluid has a green or brown tinge;
• her waters break and the baby's head had not descended properly at her previous checkup;
• she loses a considerable amount of blood (saturates two sanitary napkins within ten minutes); or
• she feels anxious.

If none of the above applies, she can wait to call her midwife or obstetrician until the contractions intensify and occur every three to five minutes for half an hour.

guests and should adapt themselves to her environment. The presence of a friend or relative can give her a sense of security and help distract her from the pain. But if at any point during the birth a woman prefers to have more privacy, she must feel free to ask guests to leave. If the possibility of this happening has been discussed ahead of time, those attending will understand and will be happy to accommodate her wishes.

A WOMAN'S SENSE of being the director of her own delivery can be disturbed easily. One of the midwife's tasks is to prevent anything from interfering with a woman's emotional and physical states. A delivery will go more smoothly in peaceful surroundings. Animals search for a sheltered place in which to give birth; women have a similar nest-making urge. When an animal is bearing young, the contractions cease if she has to flee. The contractions do not resume until peace has been restored and it is safe for her to have her litter. The human body reacts much the same way. When a woman is ill at ease or her concentration is disrupted, the contractions become less intense and may even stop. Being tense, afraid, or cold stimulates the release of adrenaline, a hormone that readys the body to defend itself. Adrenaline counteracts oxytocin, and thereby reduces the effectiveness of the contractions. Consequently, delivery is prolonged needlessly, posing additional risks for mother and child. Disturbances, which at other times would be considered inconsequential events—a wrong word, a rough touch, a door slamming, can upset the delicate emotional equilibrium of a woman during contractions. An uncomfortable position or a ringing phone can cause irritation when she is trying to give in to what is happening in her body. Simple steps, such as closing the curtains and unplugging the phone, can prevent potential disruptions.

Most often, a woman's home is where she'll feel most comfortable when giving birth; however, some women feel safer and more comfortable delivering in a hospital. If a woman prefers to have her baby

Vertical Delivery in a Hospital

HOSPITALS HOUSE MANY resilient bacteria. Because a woman is in a foreign environment, her body has not had a chance to build up resistance to these potential sources of infection. The delivery room floor is probably not hygienic because so many people move in and out of the room during the birth. Therefore, the hospital floor is unsuitable for vertical deliveries, and it is necessary to use a small platform to provide a sanitary foundation for the birthchair. Only the woman and her partner go onto the platform, and the midwife or doctor sits in front of them.

in a hospital or has a medical condition that requires her to do so, she should study the hospital's regulations so she can follow her wishes within those limitations. Some hospitals allow a woman to walk in the corridors or to take a hot shower during the contractions. She may wish to bring a table lamp from home in case the bright overhead lighting bothers her.

COPING WITH CONTRACTIONS

The intense physical and emotional experience of working hard to deliver a child cements the tie between mother and infant. To eliminate physical sensation often has an alienating effect on the woman and her baby. Needless to say, the use of anesthetics is indispensable in some situations, but the majority of women do not require medical intervention. Giving birth can be more fulfilling when natural methods such as the following are used for coping with the pain.

BREATHING: When a woman holds her breath, she may experience temporary cramping. Breathing regularly helps her deal with the strong sensations of dilatation. She will attain her own particular breathing pattern to which she can cling during a contraction. She should breathe in a manner that comes naturally to her, as exaggerating her breathing by inhaling or exhaling too deeply might cause her to hyperventilate.

POSITIONS: Certain positions, which are called active positions, make contractions easier and more effective. During the initial contractions, many women feel inclined to walk. As dilatation proceeds, we recommend that women reduce movement and assume an active position because too much muscle activity stimulates adrenaline, which can prolong delivery. The positions illustrated here assist the womb in its movements and improve blood flow through the placenta as well as being soothing for the woman during labor.

MASSAGE: Massaging the lower back, pelvis, and thighs eases pain and tension. Sometimes exerting steady pressure in those areas also brings relief.

HOT-WATER BOTTLE: The pressure from the baby's head and shoulders in the birth canal and the stretching of ligaments of the uterus cause discomfort in the lower back and stomach. Placing a hot-water bottle on the sore areas can help tremendously.

SHOWER OR BATH: Warm water relaxes the woman in labor, increases the effect of contractions, and relieves pain. Most women enjoy having contractions in warm water but prefer to leave the tub or shower during the pushing stage. A warm bath can be a very effective way to speed up cervical dilatation. In fact, dilatation advances so quickly that unexpected underwater deliveries have occurred (*see* Influence of Water, page 45). When a woman's contractions are in full swing, she can sit down in a tub of thoroughly clean hot water. (Note: If a woman's waters have broken but dilatation has not yet begun, she can take a shower but should not sit in a bath.) Water makes a woman feel freer and lighter,

making it easier for her to surrender to the final, most difficult contractions of cervical dilatation. In a bathtub, she can lie full-length on her back or on her side, letting her arms and legs float. In the shower, a woman may want to sit on a stool and have her feet resting in a footbath.

PUSHING

The next phase, the pushing, begins with the pushing urge, which women describe as an irresistible urge to bear down. Women often say they feel they can finally contribute actively to the birth when pushing begins. After hours of dealing with cervical dilatation, pushing comes as a relief. But pushing also means hard work. A woman may get discouraged if there is no visible progress after half an

What to Do If the Child Arrives Before the Midwife or Obstetrician

SOMETIMES A CHILD's birth literally takes a mother by surprise. Although births so sudden occur quite infrequently, multiparous women run a higher risk of being unprepared than do first-time mothers. In the rare event a woman's delivery progresses this quickly, there is little cause for alarm as such deliveries usually proceed smoothly.

When a woman feels that her baby is determined to arrive, she should push gently. Once the infant is born, his or her mouth and nose should be cleaned carefully, if necessary, and then the baby should be laid on its side so mucous can drain from his or her mouth. It is important that the newborn be kept warm. *Never attempt to cut the umbilical cord.* This can wait until the doctor or midwife arrives. If the cord is cut by someone without experience, the danger of infection is great.

hour of pushing and may worry that her vagina is too narrow for the baby to ever come out. At such a moment, visualizing the baby's head gaining way down the birth canal with each contraction can be helpful.

A woman may feel persistent pain due to the pressure of the head on the pelvic floor and the wall of the vagina. Tremendous pressure builds up in the pelvic floor

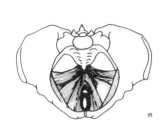

Pelvic floor muscles viewed from above

muscles because the baby's head slowly stretches them and eventually pushes them aside. The less tense muscles are, the easier they are stretched and the less pain is felt. When squatting, the gluteus maximus, a muscle in the buttocks, is stretched away from the body. Squatting allows more space around the levator ani, the most important muscle of the pelvic floor, which stretches readily in this position.

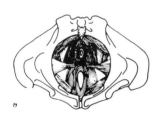

Pelvic floor muscles viewed from below

As discussed previously, the birth canal is at its widest when a woman is in a squatting position, and every millimeter counts at this point. A woman may want to change her position during the pushing, alternating between squatting, standing, kneeling, or crawling. Besides offering some variety, switching positions improves the blood flow to her lower body. Another option is the birthchair.

During the pushing, it is also important for the perineum, the area between

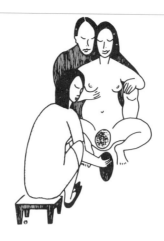

the vagina and anus, to be relaxed, and squatting produces such relaxation. Keeping the perineum warm so the muscles become pliant relaxes it even more. Between dilatation contractions or during

the pushing, a warm, wet cloth can be pressed against the perineum and the entrance to the vagina. Women find the heat soothing. The midwife can judge how far the head has descended into the birth canal by how much the perineum bulges; as the head comes down, it is necessary for her to have a good view of the perineum. By placing a mirror under the perineum, she can monitor the vaginal entrance as it is pushed open slowly. The woman and her partner can also follow the developments in the mirror.

When a woman is supine, the baby's weight pushes on the back portion of the perineum. Consequently, excessive pressure builds up in the anal region. In a vertical position, the baby's weight shifts forward in the direction of the pubic arch;

The Birthchair

A WOMAN WHO PUSHES much longer than ten minutes may find she requires more support than that which her partner can provide. The additional support of the birthchair is especially helpful for women delivering their first child, during which the pushing generally takes longer than with subsequent deliveries.

Although birthchairs in one form or another have been used throughout history (*see* History, page 3), in the recent past, a small bucket was used to support the woman while she squatted. Now a specially designed birthchair is available to facilitate the position. Birthchairs are manufactured from material that can be easily cleaned, and a stainless steel pan with a scale reading to catch and measure blood and amniotic fluid slips into the bottom of the chair's base. In order to prevent restriction of pelvic dynamics, the chair is low and shaped like a horseshoe. The upper thighs and outer portion of a woman's bottom rest on the lip of the birthchair. Excellent support is provided, which reduces the problem of the legs getting sore or falling asleep, while at the same time the tailbone and perineum remain unconfined. The woman has considerable freedom of movement. The chair has no back and no leg- or armrests, so no particular position is imposed on the woman as she sits. The "adjustable back," her partner who sits behind her, supports her as she wishes. The partner's head is close to the woman's, making it

easy for talking. This intimacy creates a sense of security. Between contractions, she can lean back and rest in her partner's arms or can get up to stretch her legs or can lower herself from the chair and kneel. During the final pushing contractions, as the head begins to show, the birthchair is usually removed; however, a woman can continue to sit on the chair while the child is born.

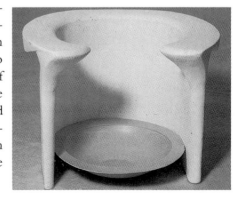

therefore, the perineum becomes less vulnerable. This shift in weight explains the reduced number of perineal tears and episiotomies (an incision made in the perineum and vagina) with vertical births; however, small labial tears do occur more frequently when the woman is upright. Such tears are often superficial, heal practically without scarring, and do not cause women discomfort during intercourse for up to six months after the delivery as is often the case with episiotomies. When perineal tears do occur in a vertical delivery, there can be considerable blood loss, most likely due to gravity. This problem is solved temporarily by having the

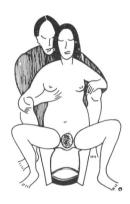

woman sit on an obstetric pad after delivery to stop the bleeding.

On its way to the outside world, the baby has to turn a corner underneath the pubic arch. Due to gravity, this takes place more swiftly and smoothly in a vertical delivery. When the head has passed the barrier of the pubic bones, the pressure on the vagina increases and the head will soon be in sight. Once the head is presented in the vertical delivery, it does not retract, disappearing between contractions a number of times, as is usually the case in supine deliveries. At this stage, following the midwife's instructions is vital for preventing tears. After the head crowns, pushing actively is no longer necessary; in fact, women are encouraged to pant, which slows the passage of the head, so the vagina is stretched gradually. In gen-

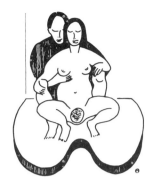

eral, a woman who listens to her body can tell that she must slow the delivery, for if she doesn't, she will have a stinging, burning sensation in her vagina. All that is required for the baby's head to be born is for the woman to sigh. Many times, with one more gentle push, the rest of the child emerges into the hands of the midwife, who lays the infant on the obstetric pad so mother and child can enjoy their first contact in their own way. The woman may sink to her knees or sit down on the pad with her child. Immediately, she sees the child's gender and whether her baby is all right. Then she can adjust to the new situation at her own pace, picking up the newborn when she feels ready.

Afterbirth

The uterus will contract after the child is born, causing the placenta and membranes to further disengage from the uterine wall and be born. This event is called the afterbirth. If a woman feels anxious about the placenta's arrival, her stress may disturb the process. Studies indicate that the intense emotions of the first contact between mother and child induce secretion of the hormone oxytocin, which increases the intensity of uterine contractions. Often while she is engaged with her baby, a woman will have contractions or a slight pushing urge, signs that the placenta is on its way.

Giving birth to the placenta entails loss of blood. To prevent excessive bleeding, it is crucial that the uterus continue to contract strongly so the broken vessels in the wall are tightly constricted. The contractions that follow the child's birth are called afterpains. The loss of blood just after a vertical delivery may seem to be rather heavy; due to gravity, amniotic fluid and blood leave the body almost immediately. This should not alarm the woman as it is actually advantageous. When blood leaves the uterus without delay, contractions are more effective, which decreases further bleeding and causes the placenta to be delivered faster. We recommend that the woman sit on a birthchair so the blood and placenta can be collected and measured in the pan at its base. In the supine position, blood stays within the uterus until the placenta is born, which sometimes takes a few minutes longer to occur than with a vertical delivery.

In addition to helping decrease blood loss, afterpains assist the womb in its return to prepregnancy size. Women often have afterpains when they breastfeed because breast stimulation releases oxytocin, which, in turn, causes uterine contractions. The womb of a multiparous woman, a woman who has delivered more than one child, is less elastic than that of a first-time mother. With each delivery, the womb's ability to return to its original size decreases. This loss of elasticity explains why multiparous women often have more intense afterpains and for a longer period of time—up to three to four days after the birth.

Following the afterbirth, the midwife checks the perineum and vagina for tears that may have occurred during the delivery. A severe tear or an episiotomy must be repaired. The area is sensitive now, but the woman is given a local anesthetic. A minor tear will heal of its own accord and does not require stitches. After the vaginal area is checked, mother and child can continue their first contact.

BEEKE

Beeke: Sylvester's mother
Sylvester: first child, a boy (born at home)
Gert-Paul: Sylvester's father
Wilma: girlfriend
Jolanda: maternity nurse
Beatrijs: midwife

THIS INTERVIEW TOOK PLACE THREE MONTHS AFTER SYLVESTER'S BIRTH.

One of the things that struck me about your delivery was that you had invited your girlfriend to be there. What was that like?

BEEKE: I thought it would be fun to ask Wilma. The fact that she had studied medicine was reassuring to me. Later, I also asked her boyfriend, who is a doctor. Another friend suggested that it might be too much to be surrounded by so many people, but I had the feeling they would be of help to me, especially because they are both in the medical field.

Were they helpful?

Yes. At a certain moment when I was in the shower, during the last part of the cervical dilatation, I really was struggling. Wilma was showering me, and she said, 'Every contraction serves a purpose,' which helped a lot.

Was this your first pregnancy?

Yes, I was afraid that I wouldn't be able to do it. I am not the sporty type, so I really exercised while I was pregnant. I paid a lot of attention to exercising my pelvic floor muscles. Perhaps it paid off because I didn't tear.

You delivered vertically. Did you do any special exercise to prepare yourself, like squatting, for instance?

I did squat with my legs spread apart to train the muscles of the pelvic floor, but I am naturally good at squatting.

Did the delivery go as you expected?

It might have been worse, especially the third stage, but seeing what was happening in the mirror helped.

You had most of your dilatation contractions in the shower. Was that the most comfortable place? Did you try other things as well?

I was lying in bed when Beatrijs arrived. I was freezing and did not feel like getting up. She suggested that I take a hot shower. If she hadn't, I probably would have stayed in bed and felt even more miserable.

Was warmth important?

Yes, and so was standing up! During a contraction, Gert-Paul helped me lower myself onto the bucket.

Did you use any breathing techniques?

I did sigh, not as was taught during the course I took, but the way Wilma had instructed to prevent hyperventilation. She taught me to breath out more slowly.

How were the pushing contractions?

In the pregnancy course, they teach you that you really have to make the most of a pushing contraction. At the beginning, I felt tired from taking a shower, and for awhile I thought, 'Just let it come'.

Was it difficult to sigh during the final contractions?

You often hear women say that, but it wasn't hard for me. Sighing is important to help slow down the delivery—especially in the vertical position where everything happens faster anyway—otherwise, you tear.

In the process of delivering did you think about and feel a connection with your child?

Most of the time I didn't. I was too involved with my own body until the end, when I could see the hair. I really like that black hair! What's so miraculous is that the vagina can turn into such a huge opening that a head can pass through.

What was it like when Sylvester came out?

The last part of the delivery was funny. As the head descends bit by bit, you get used to it; but the last part is a flood, a warm rush that flows out of you, which is wonderful and incomprehensible.

Did you pick up Sylvester, or was he handed to you?

The baby was lying on the floor. At first I just watched him. Beatrijs said, 'You can pick him up if you want,' but it wasn't that simple because Gert-Paul was still holding me under the arms. Once I was sitting on the floor, I picked him up and put him on my legs. I drew up my knees so I had a good view of him. His eyes were wide open. This struck me as odd because I had imagined a child with closed eyes which wouldn't open for some time.

Did Sylvester cry?

Yes, shortly after he had popped out. Of course, it was a rather chilly transition for him.

What made him quiet down?

I think he felt the warmth of my body as I picked him up. Then he was comfortable and warm again, and we watched him as he watched us. It was so sweet to feel his little foot touch my nipple.

How was the afterbirth?

I had forgotten all about it because I was involved with the baby. It took only a little pushing. Beatrijs pushed my stomach to help it come out.

Having a baby changes the rhythm of your life. What's that like?

I must say I was rather tired. I missed a night of sleep the night I delivered, and I didn't sleep enough the next night. Every three hours I changed his diapers and I had to pee. I was lucky to have Jolanda as my maternity nurse. She was more dedicated to mother and child than to housekeeping. In the beginning, it was one big party. Many visitors came by, so after ten days, I still felt worn out. One day, I was so tired that I dreaded having to bathe the baby. Jolanda suggested that I take the baby to bed with me after feeding him, but I was simply too exhausted to listen then.

People should be careful not to intervene too much because they can talk you into feeling like you're not a good mother. They should realize that some things do not run smoothly in the beginning. For instance, the milk does not always come in immediately. I though it would just flow. Then, I had a slight fever due to temporary congestion from too much milk. At night, I put ice cubes on my breasts, which were sensitive for four or

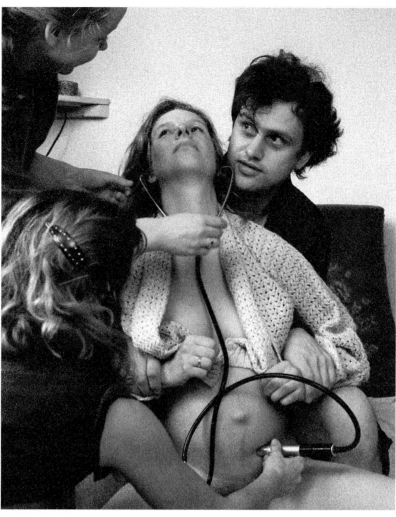

five days. I never dreamt that breastfeeding could be so painful. At first, I was not very good at it, which was trying at night. I worked out a more comfortable position, using one pillow to support my back and putting one on my lap. Now I don't need them. In the beginning, Sylvester couldn't suck very well; he sucked his own tongue rather than my nipple. I was intent on breastfeeding him, and Jolanda helped me learn how. She took my nipple with her hand, pushed down Sylvester's tongue, and inserted the nipple into his mouth properly. Once he had hold of the nipple, it went all right.

What is the difference between interacting with a baby and an adult?

First, the fact that the child is yours. You can never claim an adult to be yours,

and, in a way, you can do so with a baby. I have a greater understanding now for mothers who have trouble accepting the fact that children grow up and lead their own lives. Letting go must be painful because one image of your child that you will always carry with you is him or her as a baby. For awhile, you are constantly surprised that this child came out of you, which makes you look at your baby differently than you would any other person. The innocence and helplessness of my baby still moves me, and his total dependence frightens me sometimes. During the first months, contact with the baby is predominantly physical. The first smile is very special. A little recognition for which you've worked weeks on end. In the beginning, he was just a cuddly toy, but with that smile we established real contact with each other.

Did Sylvester look at you immediately after he was born?

Yes, but I had no idea how he was feeling. Now that he can smile, I know when he is happy.

What is so special about having your own child that you would do anything for him or her?

You may compare it to being in love, when everything in the garden is lovely. Loving the child is easy, but I don't believe people who claim that they haven't had any problems. Your child changes every week—appreciating more, seeing more, being able to do more and to start enjoying life. That's unbelievable!

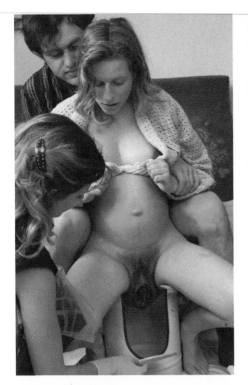

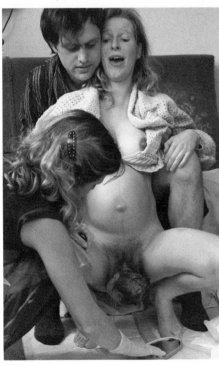

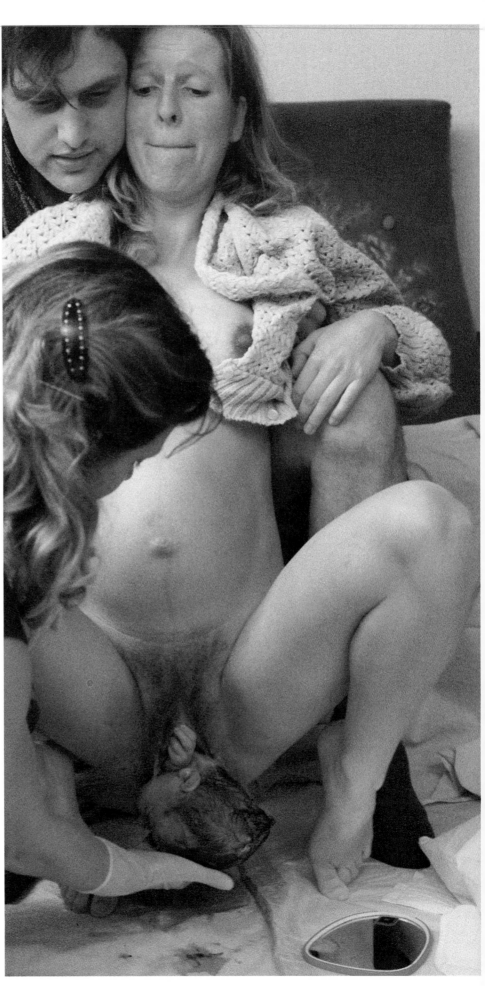

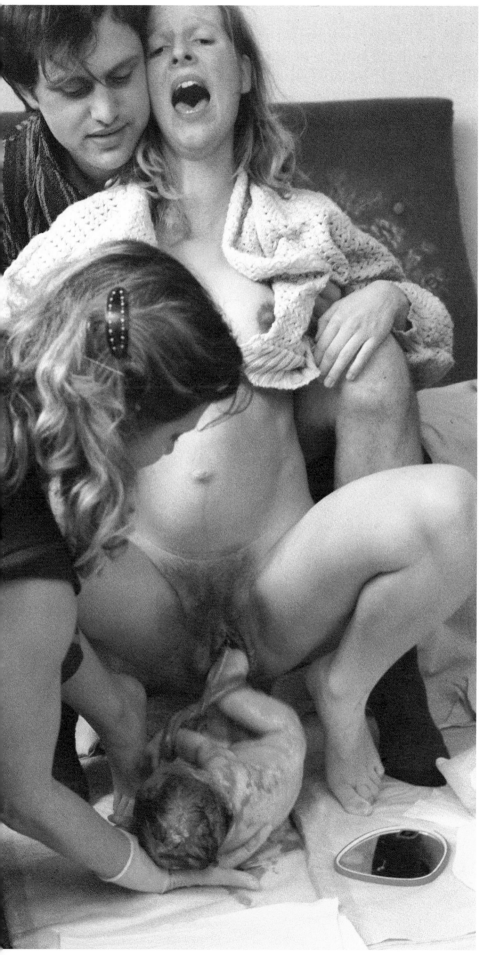
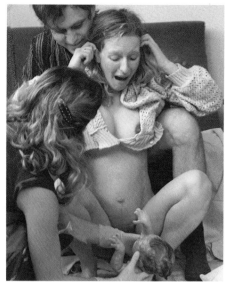
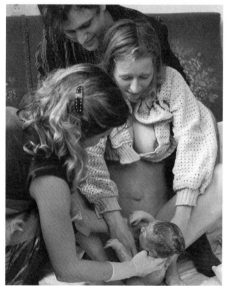
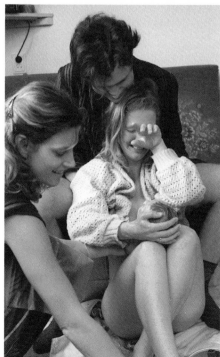

MARION AND EWOUD

Marion: Jort's mother
Jort: first child, a boy (born at home)
Ewoud: Jort's father
Cecile: Marion's sister
Sylvia: lodger
Marijke: girlfriend
Astrid and Beatrijs: midwives

THIS INTERVIEW TOOK PLACE SIX WEEKS AFTER JORT'S BIRTH.

MARION: I had formed a clear idea of how I wanted the delivery to be—the atmosphere, the location (here in the living room), and the people I wanted to be present. All went as I had visualized. I had prepared myself that labor would be fairly painful and that I might not be able to deal with it and wouldn't know what to do. Yet I was never afraid. I recall being in such great pain during my periods that I didn't know where to turn. I had imagined the pain of the delivery might be similar, but more prolonged. Even taking that into account, I wasn't scared.

EWOUD: I had expected it wouldn't be easy for Marion to find a comfortable position during the contractions, but that wasn't the case at all. She sat quietly in her chair here. All went well.

You had invited some friends. Why was that?
MARION: It just happened. We didn't really decide upon it originally. I invited people before I had discussed the matter with Ewoud, on the condition that he approved. When we talked it over later, Ewoud appeared to be less enthusiastic.

EWOUD: Well, in the beginning it was hard to imagine what it would be like with other people present. I worried that they might inhibit me during the delivery, and that's why I was not terribly in favor of it. But they had already been invited, and as they are close friends of ours, I thought it shouldn't really be a problem. But I do consider birth a sacred event

that ought to be shared by just the two of us. I would love to have that experience once, but I enjoyed the coziness of this delivery. This way, perhaps, was less 'sacred' than I had imagined, but it was a good experience nevertheless.

MARION: I simply took it for granted that others should be present. I had always wanted to attend a delivery, but the opportunity never arose. Obviously, it was the people closest to us who were asked to be there. Sylvia is our lodger, and Marijke is a girlfriend with whom I shared my 'having a baby scheme' and who will take care of Jort one day a week. We wanted to have photographs taken and thought that it wouldn't be much fun if Ewoud had to take them himself. My sister Cecile has photographed us before, so I asked her.

Did their presence inhibit you?
MARION: Not at all. Everyone warned me that it might, but it didn't put me off. I concentrated only on myself. I'd expected that I'd really need Ewoud to help me with my breathing. I had read reports of women who got totally rattled and their partners had to help them find their breathing rhythm. We talked about this in advance, and I told him that he must help me in such and such a way. But I never needed it! Perhaps that's a pity. I was glad there were people who could distract Ewoud.

Was it embarrassing that Marion needed you less than you had been made to expect from courses and various reports?

EWOUD: It was all right because we had a difference of opinion about the breathing techniques that were taught in the course. Marion was convinced she would need these techniques as a distraction during the delivery and would want to count, wanting me to help her. I did not approve of counting. I considered it unnatural and was afraid it would disturb a natural process like giving birth.

MARION: I thought the counting would be a good distraction because I'd have to concentrate which would prevent me from surrendering too much to the pain. I could understand Ewoud's feelings, but I figured I was the one who would be faced with the pain so things should be done my way and he should assist me. I was afraid he would flatly refuse, so I told him, 'You've got to do it. Don't let me down.'

EWOUD: I agreed eventually. After all, it was Marion's delivery.

But you were relieved that counting wasn't necessary?

EWOUD: Exactly!
MARION: I recall telling Beatrijs; 'I hope it's not coming yet because I'm not completely at home with the breathing technique.' Beatrijs answered, 'You don't need it—just follow your own breathing.' At that time, I didn't believe her. In retrospect, she was right. If I hadn't had the right concentration and attitude, my efforts wouldn't have been successful. I still cannot pinpoint the factors that made it work, but I found the right position.

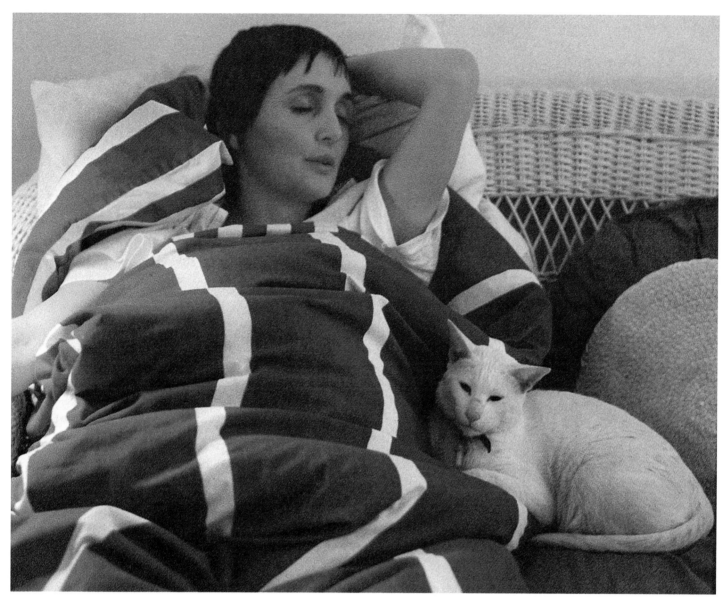

How do you feel about the pregnancy course?

EWOUD: We enjoyed the course. We gained by it, even though we had already read a lot in advance. We were introduced to calisthenics and relaxation exercises, which we couldn't do so easily on our own.

As far I was concerned, the most important purpose of the course was getting to know other people who were in the same situation and with whom we could exchange views and remain in contact. We still see some of them regularly.

What kind of relationship did you have with the midwives?

MARION: A pleasant one. You don't have a close relationship with your mid-wife instantly. I never expected that from

them. But I did enjoy the closeness once it was there. That begins to develop at the time she arrives at your house or during the delivery. Astrid conducted the delivery, after which she stayed on and chatted for a while. During the postnatal checkup everything is different than before.

EWOUD: I think a home delivery inspires a good relationship. When people come to your home, the birth is much more personal than in a hospital.

MARION: I would detest delivering in a hospital, surrounded by a whole array of people I didn't know. That was one of the main reasons I chose not to deliver in a hospital.

EWOUD: I wouldn't really object if a crowd of nurses bounced in during the prime moment of birth. But it would

bother me if friends were not allowed to be there, as is the case in many hospitals. That would be illogical.

MARION: The advantages of home delivery are clear to me. In particular, the fact that the mother determines how things are done, which is important for the course of the delivery.

EWOUD: There was quite a bit wrong with our organization.

MARION: The heater kept going out.

EWOUD: And the telephone rang at unexpected moments.

MARION: Someone called while I was pushing, which I didn't mind at all. These very ordinary events, so familiar, take away some of the pain.

Had you planned your situation carefully?

MARION: Yes, we had. I always do. But when the waters broke, things threatened to take a different course than I had planned. If the contractions don't start within twenty-four hours, you must deliver in a hospital. And that was something we hadn't considered seriously. With the exception of the Wilhelmina Gasthuis, no hospitals allowed friends to be present during the delivery. That's why we chose that hospital as a backup. But, really, at that moment I didn't care where I would deliver, I was just happy that the delivery had started. Not that the baby was overdue, but I had been yearning for it so much. I was simply impatient. I was excited that my child would arrive within twenty-four hours, and this thought consumed me.

I drank some castor oil to stimulate the contractions but couldn't bring myself to believe it would work. We went to bed. I dropped off to sleep immediately. A couple of hours later, the contractions woke me up. While Ewoud was still asleep, I counted them, registering how frequently they came and how long they lasted. I woke up Ewoud, and we went to the living room because I wanted to deliver there.

Beforehand, I had pictured myself busily walking around or doing things, but all I felt like doing was sitting quietly.

Did you sit on the sofa the whole time?

I attempted to lie down once, but that was unbearable.

EWOUD: It sometimes happens that women don't sit at all. A woman in our group, however, sat down on the toilet and refused to get off, so she just delivered on the toilet.

She was having her contractions and pushing on the toilet the way I did on the bucket. When the child emerged, her husband put himself behind her. I can understand; after all, a toilet seat is more comfortable than a bucket.

What was it like on that bucket? Was it an ordinary bucket?

EWOUD: It was a bucket with rather wide sides that flipped over. A woman from our course, who had delivered two weeks earlier, lent it to us, and she had borrowed it from yet another woman. After my delivery, the bucket went to another woman. It is a very old bucket, but it works marvelously.

To stay warm, you had a comforter wrapped around you?

MARION: During the contractions I was chilly. I craved warmth.

How did you feel when pushing?

It was hard to imagine that there really was a child. Maybe I didn't dare think about it. The fact that a child was there was somewhat eerie. I could hardly believe it, even though there was ample proof! I heard the heartbeats and could feel the baby's back and bottom, but—still—it remained inconceivable. I couldn't picture the child descending or what it would look like inside me.

I thought that focusing on the purpose of the pain would make it more tolerable, but I did not relate the pain to what was happening and to what I knew was still to come. The pain was abstract, which alienated me from my child even more during the delivery. It was odd to feel so little emotion. But when I saw the head present itself, I knew what had been causing the pain.

You could only believe it once you saw the head?

It struck me that the first time you fully realize what it means to give birth to a child is the moment it is born. You are suddenly so overwhelmed with emotions that you're temporarily at a loss. When the head presents itself, it is still something abstract. But when you feel the whole little body slide down between your legs, then you are overcome by emotion, which lasts only a minute or so. I was so overcome that I could no longer watch, so I never saw him coming out, so I regret this, but I was simply too overwhelmed.

EWOUD: I was sitting behind her and looked into the mirror and watched what others were doing at that moment. The moment the head presented itself was

overwhelming. So much happened at the same time. I got excited. At that time, I wasn't really aware how Marion was feeling. I sat behind her because I wanted to identify myself with her. And perhaps I experienced the same emotions she did at that moment. I was moved when I saw the head appearing. But I felt more deeply affected when I watched my son after he was born—he was just lying there, and Astrid cleaned his mouth and nose and asked me to cut the cord—and, also, when he was put in Marion's arms and, later, in mine.

Did he nurse immediately?

MARION: During the first days, he refused to nurse at all. He showed sucking reflexes, but he had no interest in my breast. I couldn't believe they would produce anything, either. I was worried about that. I had never leaked. But he drank the third day. It hurt tremendously in the beginning, as if he was biting my nipple.

How long did it take for your nipples to become accustomed to feeding?

At least two weeks. It still hurts now and then. The severe aching lasted a week. These days, many women tend to give up. But everyone claimed that the pain would disappear, so I was willing to persist. I never expected this pain, especially because I never wear a bra and I always go topless on the beach. I thought I had tough nipples, but this sucking is another thing altogether.

What was the first week like?

EWOUD: Awfully tiring, for me especially. I had to be host, and the maternity nurse was here only half time. Many people dropped by to congratulate us, so I had to serve coffee and cakes, which took up the first fifteen minutes of each visit. All kinds of things had to be organized. Jort had a clubfoot, so the day after he was born I had to go to the hospital, to the general practitioner, and to the insurance company. I had two days off but that certainly was not enough, so I took a few extra days off. The first days I was exhausted. I spent them washing, cleaning,

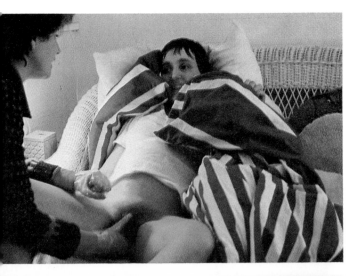

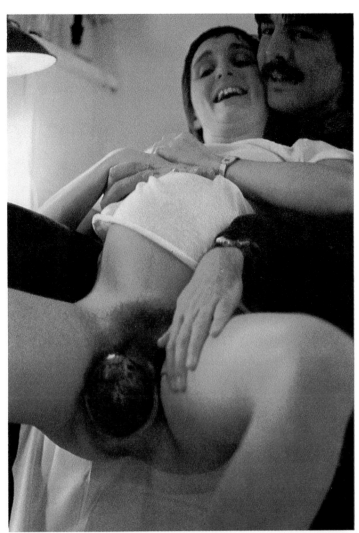

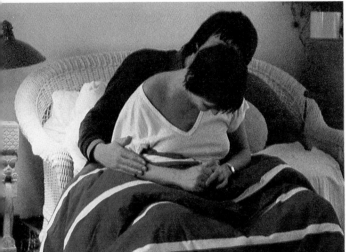

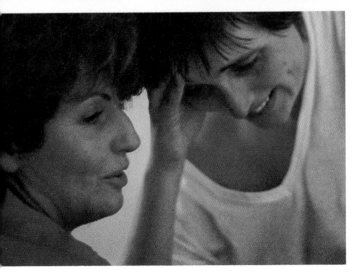

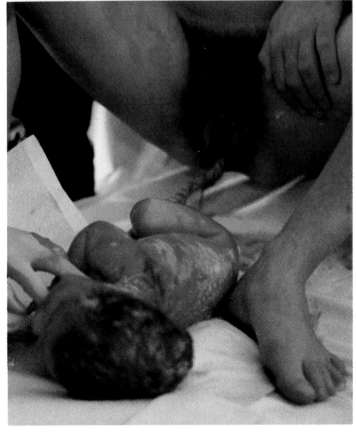

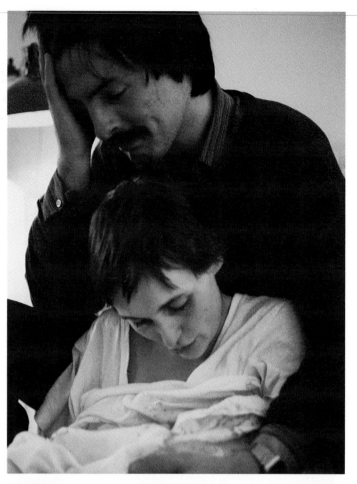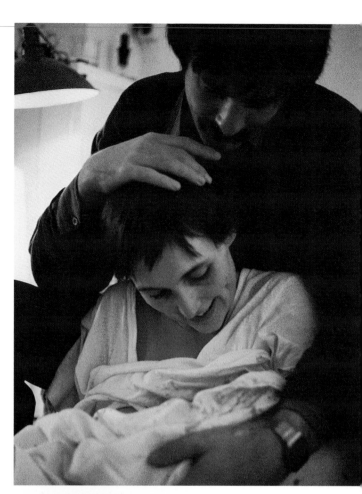
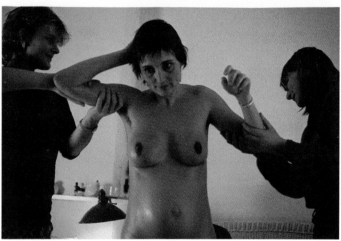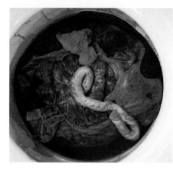

and shopping. We had put the cradle and other baby things in several different rooms of the house, which proved to be most inconvenient. We were running continually from one room to another.

Did you sleep well at night, despite Jort waking up?

EWOUD: Luckily, I can sleep very soundly, which was a pleasant discovery.

And Marion?

MARION: Jort had to be fed every two to three hours. He slept with us, on my side of the bed. We did this deliberately because we were afraid we might roll on top of him. When I push Ewoud in his sleep, he never wakes up, so he certainly wouldn't by Jort's floundering. I think changing your sleeping pattern is a matter of flipping a switch in your head. Apparently, for Ewoud this was difficult, but with me—it just happened. The first months I slept lightly, but I didn't feel less rested because of it. My fatigue during the first weeks was not caused by lack of sleep.

I had expected to have fully recovered a few days after the birth. It was quite a blow when I could do hardly anything for a week. Even when I had simply sat for an hour, I was exhausted and had to lay down. This was completely unexpected because I had had no trouble during my pregnancy and had continued working until the very end. That's why I was not prepared for the tiredness, despite the fact that everyone had warned me about it.

Why do you think you were so tired?

Probably because you've been making something in your body for nine months, which all of a sudden goes away, tipping the hormonal balance. It is not so much the delivery that causes the fatigue as the process of adapting to the altered state of your body.

That lasts a few weeks?

It took six weeks before I was my old self again.

And how long before you wanted to do things other than those involving the baby and family?

Slightly less than that. After five weeks I suddenly felt I had free time on my hands. It was only then that I could bring myself to get on my bicycle and drop in on friends. Not before that.

What about you, Ewoud? You had to go back to work after a few days, despite all the changes at home.

EWOUD: Going back to work was rather restful. That was only possible thanks to members of the family who helped Marion in the house. The transition wasn't difficult for me.

MARION: Nor for me. I still don't feel that our life has changed so drastically. It surprises me that so little has changed. The most radical change possible has taken place and yet much has remained the same. Sometimes we forget that Jort exists—less and less of course. Sometimes when we are cooking our meal in the kitchen, just as in the old days, we exclaim, 'My goodness, we've got a child here, too!'

You don't feel that you are incredibly tied down?

EWOUD: No, partly because now you can easily carry the baby in a sling. In the past you had to drag the baby carriage up three flights of stairs. This would discourage you from going out a lot.

When did you start using the sling?

EWOUD: After two weeks we went out for the first time.

MARION: It is marvelous but rather heavy. In the beginning I took him shopping with me, but really that's too taxing. Then I didn't dare go out for a long time, and bicycling with him frightened me—now I think nothing of it.

Do you take him with you wherever you go?

MARION: Yes, even to parties.

EWOUD: Often people are mildly surprised when the three of us arrive on one bicycle.

KNOES AND KARIN

Knoes: Devi's mother
Devi: second child, a boy (born at home)
Zowi: first child, two-year-old boy (born at home)
Jef: Devi's father
Karin: Knoes's girlfriend

THIS INTERVIEW TOOK PLACE THREE MONTHS AFTER DEVI'S BIRTH.

KNOES: It all started in the supermarket, butterflies in my stomach, staring at the bottles, and breathing. I had had pre-contractions before and thought these were similar. When I got home, I started preparing a meal, but I didn't really feel like eating. I took a shower. It made me feel nice and fresh. Judging from my tummy I knew this was the real thing.

I played an album, continued cutting up the food, and danced during the contractions. Finally, I called Beatrijs. I thought that she would like that.

After half an hour, the contractions followed one another every five minutes, and after that, they came reasonably fast. I didn't really want to give birth yet and was crying a little bit. I did not have the energy to cope with contractions. I sat down on the sofa and called Karin to ask her to come over.

KARIN: When we came in, you were totally involved with yourself and hardly responded to us at all.

What was that like for you? Had you seen her like that before?

KARIN: Knoes always retreats into herself when she is in pain.

KNOES: We have been friends since childhood and have gone through the roughest times together, talking together, so everything is very open. I had invited her because she is a close friend. It is enjoyable to be able to share with her what goes on inside me, for after all, it is quite a change. You go through something that is new to the other person, and you want to let her participate in it, to show her what it is like and what is happening to you, that there is a child and how you develop and change with a child in your life.

Was this the first time you've been at a birth?

KARIN: I wasn't so involved with Knoes' first delivery. I didn't think about it; I wasn't ready for it then. At a certain moment, I noticed that Zowi's birth had brought changes in Knoes' life and things were going well for her.

Then my curiosity about the delivery was aroused. I thought about it long after the delivery, and for quite some time I was shaken by it.

KNOES: It is great to be able to talk about your delivery to friends. You can share the experience, despite the fact that you've done it by yourself. During the delivery, I felt uninhibited. It doesn't matter whether you're pooping or peeing. There are no rules. You act on the spur of the moment and follow your instincts. After the delivery, a sense of shame slowly returns. The whole process is so beautiful that I wish I could experience it a hundred times.

KARIN: I had always had scary thoughts about delivering a baby: lots of blood and pain. But it was splendid.

KNOES: That is what I had also imagined it to be like—those horrible things you often hear. But when I experienced it myself, it dawned on me that giving birth was the most beautiful thing in the world. I was in pain all right, but I could cope with it easily. After that came the joy over the arrival of another child.

You didn't mind the pain?

The way people talk about birth frightened me, but in reality it wasn't dreadful at all.

Had you taken a class to practice coping with contractions?

With my first child, Zowi, Beatrijs had told me about a pregnancy course. She had given me the address, and we enrolled ourselves. You had to take your husband along, and it was so stupid at first. It scares people in the sense that they feel they must attend pregnancy classes because without them they won't be able to deliver properly. Giving birth is a natural process, something thousands of women have gone through—nothing horrifying, simply an ordinary part of life. Anyway, we went and chatted with others about how long we'd been pregnant and told each other our names and professions and God knows what else. Well, all these women with fat bellies were sitting there, and then all of us had to sigh. And then it started: first breath in deeply—and, of course, all the women were dying of laughter and then pft, pft, pft, pft, I couldn't do it for it seemed so stupid to me—and then breathing out. You simply puffed and sighed. Then we were told to lie with our backs on the floor and relax, which I found impossible, and so I instantly concluded that my delivery was going to be a fiasco. I sat there and giggled nervously.

Then Jef had to hold my foot so I

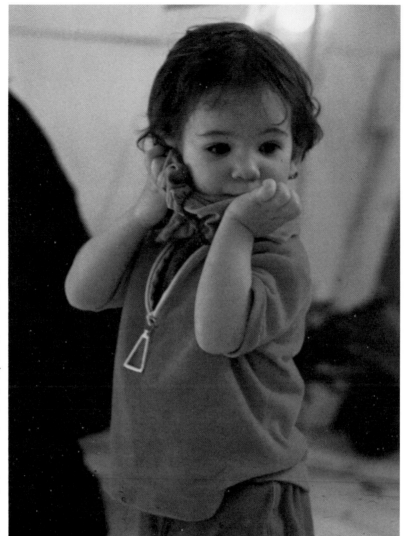

would relax, but I was tense as anything. It was too ridiculous to be true—here's my foot and here I go, relax!

The classes didn't suit us at all. We often arrived late, which was silly, of course. Anyway, I imagine that such a course is more suitable for women who dread the delivery.

Retrospectively, did you benefit at all from that course?

No, I don't think so. I am the kind of person who in certain situations acts better on instinct than with instructions. Take dancing, for instance. When I have to do a particular dance step, I'll immediately move in the wrong direction, but if I am allowed to follow my own devices, I do quite well. That's why the course was useless for me.

Do you listen to what your body tells you?

Yes, I pay attention to where the pain comes from, and I respond. When I've got a headache, I just sit down. You may call it meditation. I withdraw into myself and find peace and get myself together again.

Were things different your first delivery, with Zowi?

That delivery was much more exciting. I had no idea what to expect. I was much more nervous. At Zowi's delivery, I

kept moving my feet during a contraction because I was tired and unmotivated, and this caused me to lose my concentration. This time, I realized that I had to keep my feet on the ground and remain seated quietly without resisting the contractions. I just accepted them and didn't wish them away. It is better to surrender and think, 'Baby, how about coming out fast?' Then things go easier. Last time, we were given a chart on which we had to jot down the times of the contractions. So each time I had a contraction, I wrote it down—but only because that's what I was taught in class—which is too crazy for words.

Was Zowi born at home, too?

In the beginning, I wanted a twenty-four-hour clinical delivery because it was the first time. The stories I had heard

had frightened me. For instance, at first I believed that I was not allowed to ride a bicycle after I was three months pregnant. But then I discovered I could still do an awful lot. I bicycled and played tennis until I was nine months pregnant. These stories never get about, which is such a pity for it is great fun. I was sitting in the midwife's waiting room, and another woman told me she was going to deliver at home. She said that delivery is not an illness. I though she was right. I had dreaded the idea of calling a taxi to take me to the hospital. I despised the fact that you had to organize so much, like arranging transportation and packing the baby's clothes. For a home delivery, you don't have to worry about such things. You can wait for the moment with everything at hand.

Were friends present at your first delivery?

Yes, a girlfriend of mine was there. The three of us used to do lots together in the old days, so I appreciated her presence at the delivery.

How did you occupy yourself during cervical dilatation?

I relaxed on the sofa. I watched and I dreamed and I listened to other people's conversation. As a contraction begin, I stared at a spot on the wall. But, in fact, I was looking inside myself. Then I breathed quietly. The pressure on my anus gave the impression of something turning. I became aware of the head moving backward and then forward. I clearly felt it turning. That was beautiful. I shifted my stomach and bottom, moving with the baby. When I pushed its head very hard and moved at the same time—the contractions really hurt then—I breathed harder, too.

Then the pain slowly subsided, and I could listen to the conversation of the people around me before another contraction came on. The whole time I watched Beatrijs, who went through the contractions and breathing with me; we looked at each other, which was beautiful, as though we were both in some kind of a trance. Our eyes would meet, and nothing else existed at that moment. It made me tranquil, and she made calm movements with her hands, as if saying let it come.

And then the pain stopped again. I took less comfort from Jef, for what does he know about it and Beatrijs is the midwife. Sometimes I found a contraction hard to bear, but I came to terms with it when I looked at Beatrijs who emanated such a quiet, secure feeling.

Our contact was very good, especially during the final contractions.

Did you mind the vaginal examination?

No. I think that it accelerated the process. At a certain point during the contractions, she examined me, and it seemed as if it widened me. Her hand was inside me, and I felt that I was saving time this way. I really enjoyed it and found it relaxing.

Did you feel any connection with your baby during the contractions?

Yes, definitely. I knew the baby was about to be born and thought 'Do come out.' From the pressure, I felt quite clearly that—with lots of power and energy—something was pushing to come out. I can't really describe it as pain; it was

his power and energy in my stomach that made me puff and sigh and let off steam.

So you didn't really experience the delivery as painful?

Pain is not the right word, and the word 'pain' is frightening. With Zowi, I regretted not having written it down, because after the delivery I could give an exact description of a contraction. After a while I forgot. If people asked me, I just couldn't answer. It is similar to pain associated with having a period, because then you also have to get rid of something. It is hard to put into words.

I felt the motion, which I could not control and, therefore, had to puff it out. Normally, it is you who controls how you walk and how you breath, but this process is out of your control. That's why it takes such concentration, because this is a new feeling that you have got to become familiar with in order to handle it well.

Is birth something that happens outside yourself, something that isn't personal?

No, but there are two of you. The other person, the baby, is at work, too, and you have to solve the problem together.

Did you feel a connection with the baby during your pregnancy?

I am very levelheaded about my pregnancies, and neither time was too obsessed. I never really touched my stomach with my hand. I simply grew fatter and would sometimes comment, 'Stop that trampling, will you?' Very boorish really. At times, I imagined that I might have a handicapped child because one never knows what is in store. I fantasized about the implications of various situations.

Did you ever attempt to picture the baby in detail?

No, I didn't. Just that it was a human being with the shape of a human being, not a small pig!

Did you ever dream about the birth?

Delivery dreams? Yes, twice or so. The dreams were immensely beautiful. I

can't recall them very well, but I remember waking up thinking, 'Oh, what a lovely boy.' One time I really felt I was holding him when I woke up, and then there was nothing....Silly, isn't it? It was always a boy. At three months I threatened to miscarry, so I had an ultrasound taken. I saw the baby move and instantly remarked 'Oh, it is a boy.' It looked just like Zowi in terms of its movements, the typical movements of a boy. Really odd. Ultrasounds are marvelous. And, later, I had another one done, and the only things I saw then were bones. But at three months, I could really see him swim.

Do the movements you saw then resemble his current gestures?

Yes, they really do. The other day I pointed out to Jef, 'Look, that's how he was moving about in my stomach. Inside, he moved spasmodically. His gestures became more exuberant when he was born and he could stretch out properly. What was so lovely is that thinking about him made my breast give milk. When I thought of him, he would start to cry, but only during the first two weeks. It seems too crazy to be true! I thought 'Well, that's well organized! We're totally attuned to each other.' But this went away slowly.

Is the initial bonding more intense than that which occurs later?

Because I carried the child for nine months it was obviously there. That's why I didn't hesitate to hand him to others in the beginning. Later, when he started to smile and make sounds, there was more warmth in our contact. In the beginning it all was so new. We didn't really understand each other; physically, we did, but there was no mental connection until the laughing and the noises began. Then he started to try to tell me things and I'd think: 'What is it he needs?' And in this way the connection intensified.

Was your first delivery a vertical birth?

I was supine the first time, although I would have preferred to deliver vertically even then. I had heard of it and it was on my mind. I thought it must be com-

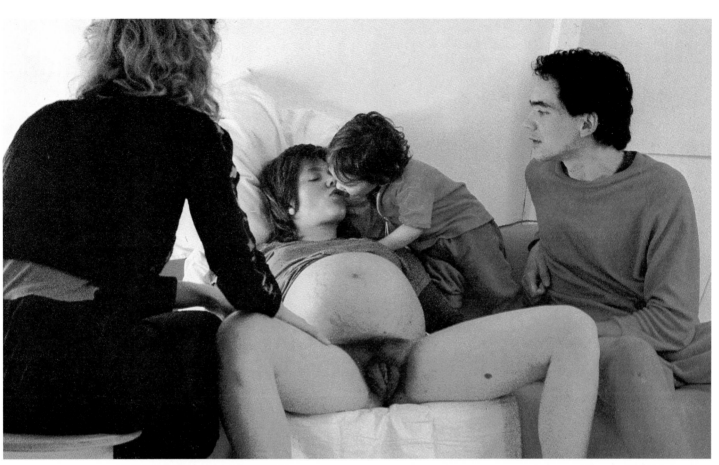

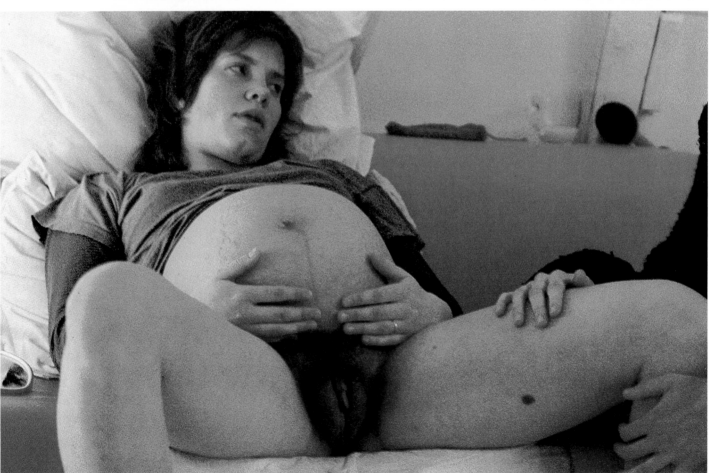

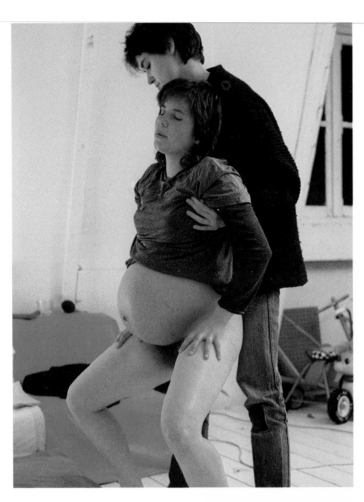
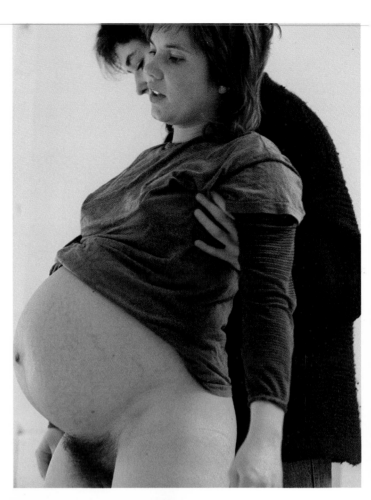
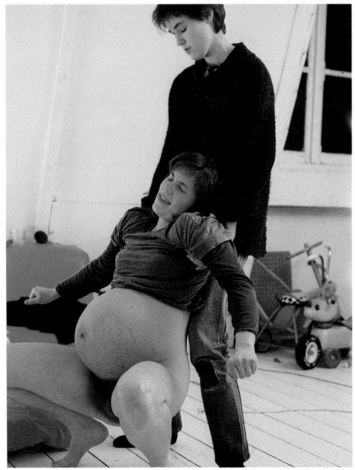

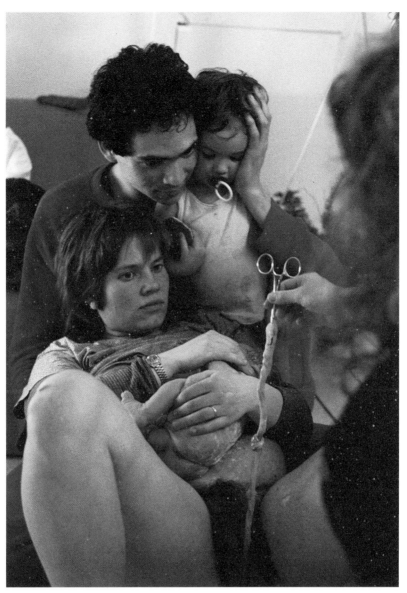

fortable. But I had a contraction and was asked to lay down for a vaginal examination and I didn't feel inclined to get up after that. I felt like lying down; I was tired and had already put in lots of effort to get up. I had no desire to do it again at that moment.

With Devi, I was sitting on the sofa initially but wanted to get up at a certain moment. It took a lot out of me—I was trembling—but once I had taken the step it was great. Being supine is heavy, everything is pressing down on you; when you are standing up, someone can support you, which is enjoyable. Standing made me feel stronger. During the pushing, I went down on my knees with such an urge and a primitive shriek. I couldn't have done that if I was lying on my back. Standing

up I could totally surrender to the pushing, and each time I made progress. During my first delivery, lying down prevented me from letting go. It seemed I was pushing for nothing. Pushing out Zowi lasted much longer, too, but this time it happened in three minutes, which was unbelievable.

People in jungles give birth this way. They hold on to a tree. It is really very logical.

Karin, was supporting Knoes hard work?

KARIN: I can't remember very well. She was heavy all right, but I only noticed that because I was trembling. But, strangely, otherwise I was not aware of it.

I regretted it when Knoes said, 'Let Jef take over.' It was going so well.

KNOES: That's true, but I felt Jef should be involved as well since he is my husband.

The idea that he could be of assistance and could help me at that moment seemed important to me.

Had you practiced how you would stand in advance?

KNOES: No, I had no idea how to do it. I asked Beatrijs when I should get up because I wanted to deliver in a standing position. But all she told me was to get up slowly when I felt like getting up. Getting up wasn't easy because I felt so feeble I had already used up a lot of energy. My legs were trembling. But I enjoyed standing. Then there was a contraction, and I wondered when to

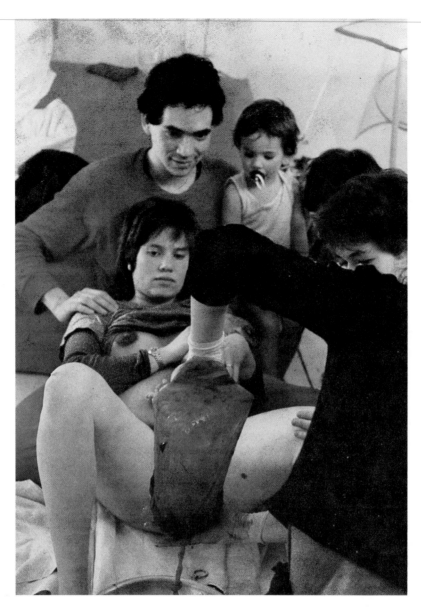

start pushing for I had no urge. Then I thought that I would just relax and I pushed and screamed and I made progress. I felt myself open up a bit and that was encouraging and exciting.

The others advised me to take things a little easier so I wouldn't tear. The urge was so powerful, however, that I feared I couldn't hold it. I heard, 'Stand up again,' and so I did, and the next time I sat down proved to be the last as the baby was born then.

Beatrijs had insisted that I take it easy and not push so hard. I tried in vain. I longed for the baby to come out. I never expected the delivery to happen so quickly and had thought I would be at it for at least another half hour. I was quite sur-

prised by Devi's sudden arrival—it was amazing.

During a delivery, you're much stronger than you think. You're very strong, in fact. I think it has to do with life and death, although this may seem sinister. You are in pain, you have to deal with the pain, and slowly but surely the pain is relieved. That's true for all things in life. It's a part of the process of life. Your mind is affected, you reach a climax, and then your child slowly emerges. You have to deal with something you can't control within your body. That's the art of giving birth.

What is it like when your child is given to you just after birth?

I am very down to earth. Devi was put on my stomach and I said, 'Oh dear, what a darling.' I remember saying this with Zowi, too, partly because it was expected of me. I thought I had to be happy now that my child had been born. But to me, the child was already born a long time ago. He had been in my stomach so long that he was already part of my life. He was alive in my belly. I had no idea what he would look like, but I was sure that he was coming. I was involved with that for nine months and suddenly he was here and I knew it was a child because what do humans do? Give birth to babies. The transition was not abrupt. The child was out, and I was busier than ever washing diapers. Things I didn't need to do when

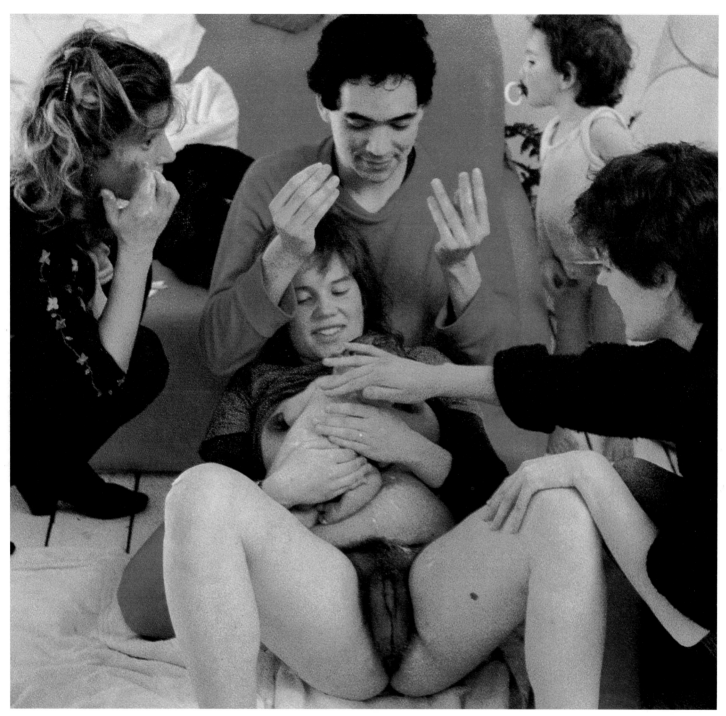

I was still carrying him inside me. I know that this is hard for a lot of women. Comforting and paying attention to your child is a lot of work and takes up a great deal of your time. You get used to it, but this is hard for some women who don't realize in advance that children are a twenty-four-hour job.

Has Zowi talked about the delivery?

He did the next morning. The delivery took place late, and he was weepy and tired. But when he woke up the next morning, he walked to the cradle and said, 'baby, baby.' That was so sweet. We had made a bed on the floor for the four of us. And then he started to talk of 'bood, bood.' He had seen the blood and mommy's belly.

In the video, you can see that he was deeply impressed by that big belly, which made him exclaim, 'Mama, big belly, big belly, look!' He also cried seeing the expressions on my face of what I was going

through. His reactions were so beautiful. I enjoyed his reactions. The birth affected him deeply, and he has talked about it long afterwards. During the contractions he cried, 'Mommy getting baby.' He understood what was going on a little bit.

He accepted Devi very well and loved to sit on my lap and cuddle him. Sometimes he wants to take him on his own lap. He's very sweet and cuddly with him and they lie in one bed. This worried me initially. Devi would be lying quietly in

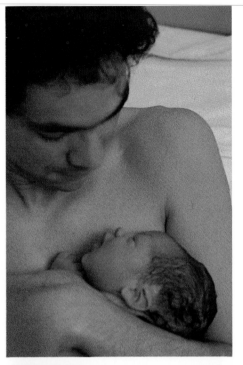
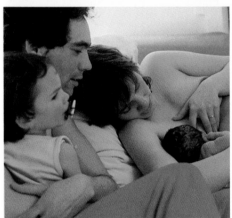
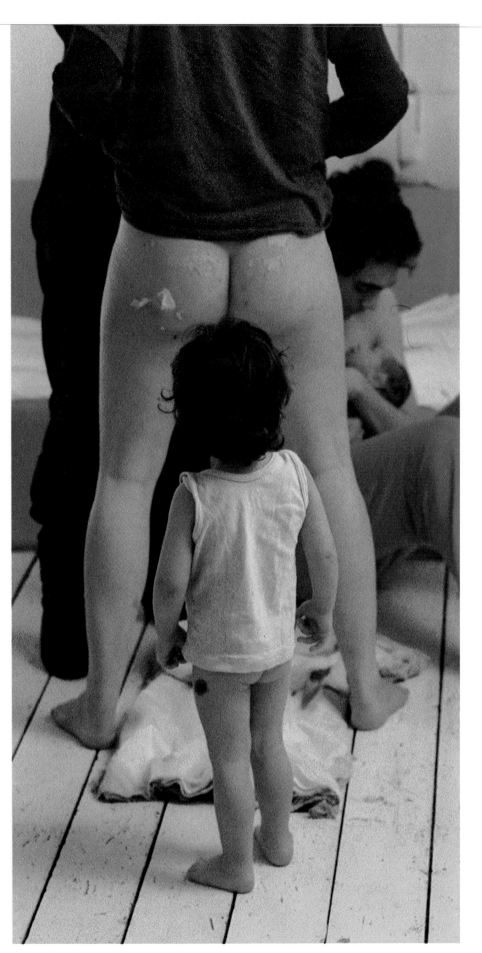

his little chair, and then Zowi would join him and be very rough. We had to teach him to be gentle. I realize that babies can stand quite a bit, but I worried he might get hurt. If I leave them to themselves, he is careful, but because I warn him time after time, he starts to play tricks.

One time I watched secretly, restraining myself from intervening, and saw that things were improving. After that, I put them in one bed, and they started to cuddle each other. When Jef and I kissed they would do the same.

What was it like for you with Zowi at the birth?

I was rather busy, you know. I couldn't really pay attention to him during a contraction. Normally, I react instantly when he utters a sound, even if I don't feel like reacting. So when I heard him, I had difficulty concentrating on what I was doing. But it was cozy to have him there, despite the distraction. If he wanted to sit on my lap during a contraction, I'd call Jef. I couldn't bear for anyone to touch me. It made me very tense.

What was the afterbirth like?

A bore because I was fed up; I had had enough. I had my child and that was enough. I wanted the placenta to be removed immediately because I knew it would all be over then, finished, no more bother. Knowing that the placenta was still inside made me restless. Then I felt something like a contraction, and Beatrijs pushed my tummy, which I hated and was most painful. I didn't feel like working on these contractions anymore; my mind was occupied with other things. I refused to concentrate again and have contractions for the mere placenta.

There was a knot in the umbilical cord. Did this upset you?

No, the child was lying on my stomach and all was well. When there is such a knot people say 'It is an owl,' a funny metaphor. So I thought, 'How wonderful, my child must be special.'

Did you have a nurse come in or did you do everything by yourself or get help from friends?

With Devi, I decided to do without the help of a maternity nurse. But it was rather hectic. I did many things I wasn't really up to. I wanted to organize all kinds of household chores like cooking, cleaning, and other little things. I wanted to do these things but didn't have my usual strength.

What is most special about the contact with such a tiny child?

First, that it comes our of your tummy and you made it together with your partner. It's a miracle, incomprehensible, really. In the beginning, I fussed over him and didn't quite know what to do with him. I know how to deal with adults, who can move, react, and express themselves. Expressions are hidden in a baby. I communicate without words. Something makes us understand each other, at least I think so, although I am never absolutely sure. I wonder what he might want. If both of us are happy, we have understood each other; if he cries, we haven't and the communication has fallen short. There are times I think we get on well together, and others when we do not pick up each other's signals. It is all so honest, so open. Nothing is disgusting. I am quite willing to catch his poos in my hand, so to speak, and that is extraordinary, because the sight of feces is usually disgusting to me. But now it is all part of the relationship. It is like stepping back into nature a bit, just as I did during the contractions when I didn't care what I looked like, what others saw, and when I felt no shame. A child has no shame, and because we went through the birth together, he and I are not ashamed of each other.

Do you feel the baby has changed your life?

Definitely. As I already mentioned, life is more hectic. I have to pay attention to my children and have less time for things. I have to divide my attention to keep track of what is happening around me. I am constantly making sure that the children don't fall down the stairs.

I simply have less time, so I can't continue my old life. It is crazy to see the children grow, to watch them play, smile, and hear them chat, to be sad with them, even to have your cry with them. These things are superb. Zowi understands when I am dejected or gloomy. I can see it in his face. He says, 'Mama cry.' I like his reaction to my bad moods—it gives me a kick. There is a mutual stimulation and that's exciting. For now I have to stimulate Devi, but when he grows up a bit he will stimulate me by laughing and playing and with his ways of enjoying himself. I learn a lot from them. Their warmth, their exuberance, their dear arm gestures fill me with drive and energy.

Is having children an experience you have always longed for?

Before I met Jef I had never slept with a boy. I was resolved not to go to bed with a man unless he would be the father of my children. Very solid, don't you agree? This came true and I am very happy about it.

We had the children. In the beginning, this scared Jef. He wasn't sure whether he was ready for it, but I certainly was. It meant a lot to me. And, at first, Jef did not want a second baby, partly because Zowi was only two years old. But, well, at a certain moment we were bungling with these condoms. We simply became lazier and then we got used to the idea of having another one and then I was pregnant.

What's so funny is that a delivery takes only a few hours of your whole life and yet so much happens that you never experience again. If you think about it, it is so odd that one day, one day of your life, has such an effect. A new life is born and that's the most beautiful thing imaginable.

MARLIES AND RINUS

Marlies: Sjoerd's mother
Sjoerd: first child, a boy (born at home)
Rinus: Sjoerd's father
Mrs. Timmermans: midwife

THIS INTERVIEW TOOK PLACE THREE WEEKS AFTER SJOERD'S BIRTH.

When did you decide not to deliver in the supine position?

MARLIES: At the pregnancy course they inquired whether you preferred the vertical or the supine position. Only one other woman and I wished to deliver vertically.

You delivered on your knees. What was that like?

I had heard that this position is very intimate and it proved to be so because Rinus and I were facing each other and I could put my arms around him. I was not aware of the people around me. This was pleasant, but I wonder whether another position might have involved me even more with the birth and the child.

You were in the middle of remodeling your home during your pregnancy and had really worked to get it finished so you could deliver at home. The bath was ready and you stayed in it quite a while during labor. What was it like to be bathing during the contractions?

Mrs. Timmermans arrived fairly late. I had already had somewhat of an urge to push. She examined me immediately upon arrival and concluded that my cervix had dilatated eight centimeters. She suggested that I get into the tub. She massaged my tummy with a hot shower, which was lovely as the last contractions were rather painful.

Being in the bath relaxed me and loosened me up. Had she arrived earlier, I would have gotten into the bath sooner. I was quite keen on delivering there as well, but the bathroom itself was too chilly.

How did you deal with your contractions?

Badly. Now I would go about it completely differently. At the pregnancy course, they talked of the ten breaths, the eight, six, four, and then the two breaths. All these different techniques were very confusing, and I never really fully under-

stood them. I did ask once when to apply which technique, but the answer was, 'You will find out when the time comes.' You start with ten and then you go down to two. I was at two very rapidly and hyperventilated slightly. Mrs. Timmermans breathed with me while I was sitting in the bath. This helped and was relaxing.

Your parents were present at the delivery. What was that like?

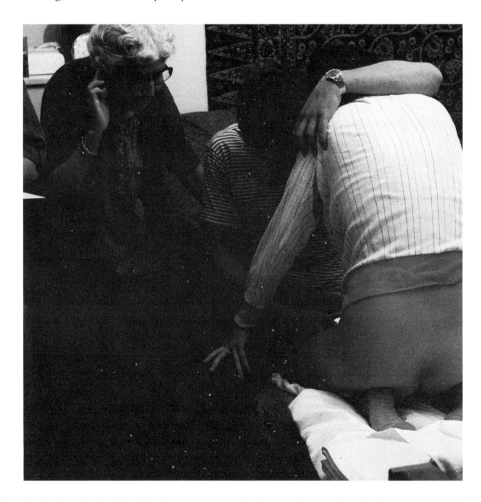

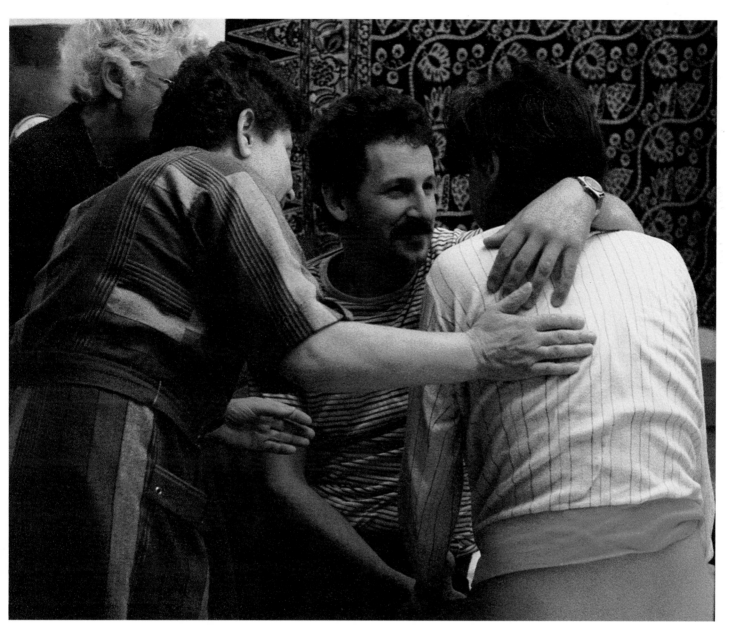

It worked out well because they distracted me a little. My parents had been slightly wary because they thought there would be screaming and more pain.

What did your mother think of your delivery?

She enjoyed it and would do it again. Initially, my father was scared, but he was also delighted. Whenever I see them now, they talk about it. The birth really has made a tremendous impression on them. A lot depends on the kind of relationship you have with your parents or with your friends. I would have been pleased if a girlfriend had been there, too. During a contraction, I was totally turned in on myself, but as soon as it subsided, I became

aware of my surroundings again. I would chat away until the next contraction, at which point everyone ceased to talk while I squeaked for a few moments. Then we would continue our conversation where we left off. They gave me a lot of moral support.

Was the pain like you imagined?

Not really. From six months on I had precontractions. Mrs. Timmermans used to say that I was too active. These contractions occurred some thirty-odd times a day. I thought the real contractions would be like that, but stronger. But they were more intense than I ever imagined.

Were you conscious of the moment of complete cervical dilatations?

No.

But you felt a pushing urge?

Yes, I did in the bath, but the cervix was not entirely dilatated then. I was allowed to push a little when the urge came. Later, on my bed, when I was on my knees, I started to push.

Did it seem as though it was a human being that was about to come out of you? Could you picture it?

Something alive, though not a real human being. I had seen pictures and photographs of birth in books, which I

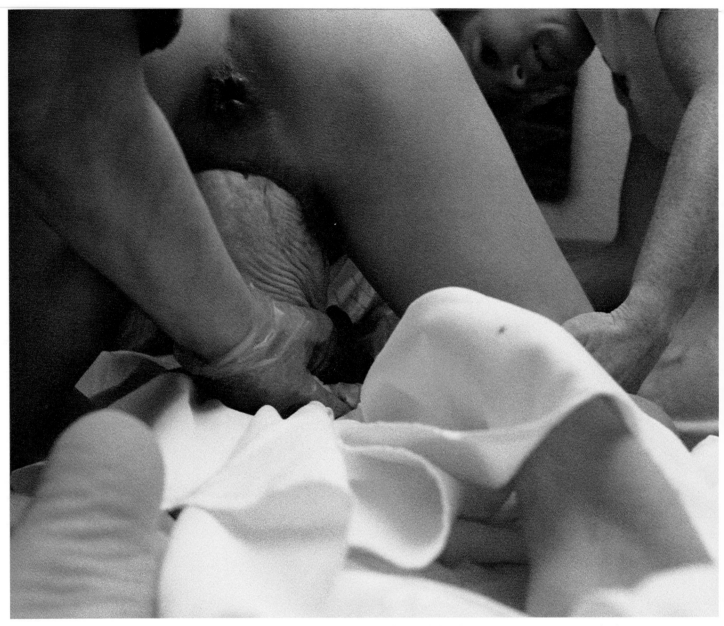

enjoyed reading when I was pregnant. But when Sjoerd came out and was lying underneath me, I was shocked that he had emerged from me. I was perplexed about that fact for a few days after the delivery.

Did you actually feel him coming out?

Yes, it was stupendous. The head had presented itself and the stretching was hurting a lot. I was told to push one more time, but I lacked the strength. Then I felt something warm and slippery slide out.

You couldn't see the baby?

No, the midwife pushed him toward me with her hand while I was still kneeling. I watched him for awhile; I did not feel like picking him up. The umbilical cord fascinated me because I had never seen a color photograph of one. Its color surprised me: a very beautiful greenish blue. Only then did it hit me that I had to do something with him, so I picked him up.

Did Sjoerd respond to you?

I was not aware of it. I noticed there was contact between Sjoerd and Rinus. I held him at my breast for a few moments. Subsequently, the placenta emerged, sliding out in the same way that Sjoerd had. It was quite a mass. Then Sjoerd was given to me again, but a blood clot had remained behind, and it hurt terribly when Mrs. Timmermans pushed it out. I got a headache after that.

Do you have an explanation for that?

Perhaps it was the tension, the exertion, or maybe it was caused by the injection to stop the bleeding. That seems reasonable because it came on suddenly and stayed on for one day and one night. I had to vomit all the time, even though my stomach was empty. I took no notice of Sjoerd. Luckily, Rinus cared for him. At the pregnancy course, I heard stories about husbands who were very involved with the pregnancy, making pictures and so forth, but Rinus was never like that. At first I regretted that, but I shook off those feelings. Sometimes people get talked into something that they are not interested in, so you have to remain aware of your own needs and desires. But from the moment Sjoerd arrived Rinus changed diapers and chatted to him all the time while I watched from my bed with astonishment.

What did you do with the placenta?

I buried it in the garden and planted a pear tree over it.

Do you feel that your relationship with Sjoerd has improved over these past few weeks?

Yes, perhaps because I feel rested and because he reacts to me now. He watches me constantly. When he hears my voice, he turns his head toward me. I notice that he reacts to my calling him nowadays.

What is most special about having a child?

That he is such a tiny creature and that everything works. I do not feel that he is mine, not that that was my reason for having a child. The other day someone commented that having a baby gives you a purpose in life and improves the relationship with your husband. This does not apply to me. I have always had a purpose in life. And if having a child is used as a means to improve the parents' relationship, the relationship is not good in the first place.

Did pregnancy and birth influence your relationship with Rinus?

I just know that we are both terribly exhausted! At night, all we can do is give each other a quick, little kiss. It has not deepened our relationship, which was already deep.

Do you behave differently now that you have a child?

When I talk to Sjoerd, I talk differently—much the same way that I adapted my speech when I taught kindergarten.

And you, Rinus?

RINUS: I think I have changed the way I talk, too. The sound is more important than the words you actually say. The child within you emerges again.

When you two talk about the birth and having this child, do you feel you share the experience or did you experience it differently than Marlies?

We have not discussed it very much. It just happened, and we are very happy with it.

Can you remember your first impressions?

I will never forget them. The birth really moved me, which I hadn't expected.

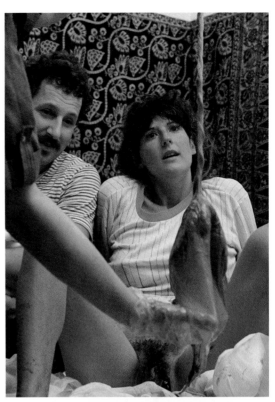

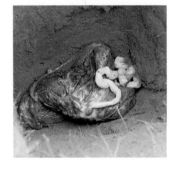

What is it like to feed him at night?

MARLIES: I have adjusted my sleeping by now. Sunday night, for instance, he did not call, but I kept waking up every three to fours hours anyway. When he does not feed, I can really feel my breasts swell. When he starts to cry I think, here we go again, but the moment I take him out of his cot, looking so sweet, my heart melts.

Has giving birth changed you?

The delivery was quite an experience in itself. I felt strong after the delivery in the sense that I felt like nothing could happen to me anymore. I don't believe you experience this at any other point in your life, unless you survive a terrible accident. When you give birth, you are between life and death, a feeling that cannot be compared to anything else.

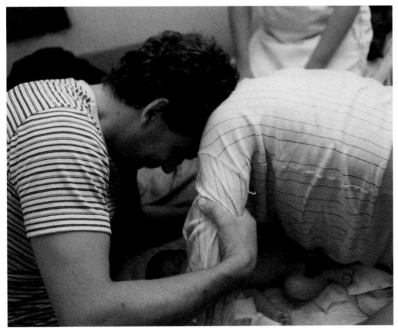

MENA AND TON

Mena: Florian's mother
Florian: first child, a boy (born at home)
Ton: Florian's father
Agaath: midwife

THIS INTERVIEW TOOK PLACE TWO MONTHS AFTER FLORIAN'S BIRTH. MENA AND TON CONDUCTED MOST OF THE DELIVERY THEMSELVES BEFORE AGAATH ARRIVED.

Both of you are medical students. Did your training influence how you handled the birth of your child or did you feel naive?

TON: Although I never applied what I had learned consciously, it was in the back of my mind.

Was the birth different from what you had expected from reading medical texts?

TON: Not really, but I have had very little clinical experience yet so my image of birth was very abstract.

MENA: You can learn medical textbooks by heart, but I think I learned more from my own pregnancy than from medical school.

Had you tried to imagine what the delivery was going to be like?

Certainly, I had fantasized about all kinds of possible situations, and how to act accordingly. But things turned out differently than I had expected.

MENA: I had heard other women talk about their experiences but had never clearly imagined what my situation would be like.

Did you dread the delivery?

MENA: A bit. Luckily, I had not imagined the pain; I thought it was not going to be painful. I dreamed three times that things would go smoothly. In these dreams, everything happened very fast—exactly as it did in fact happen. No midwife was present in my dreams; I always did it by myself. I never expected that this would happen in real life.

Labor began much sooner than you expected, didn't it?

Yes, and very suddenly. The waters broke when I went to the bathroom. I didn't even notice, so I just went back to bed until the contractions became too intense for me to remain there. I woke Ton when I thought it was getting serious.

TON: We had calculated the due date so, at first, we did not realize that the birth was about to happen. Oddly enough, both of us had dreamed that the child would be born prematurely, but, at that moment, it never crossed our minds that it was time.

At what stage did you call your midwife?

Ton called Agaath when he realized what was happening. She arrived at four o'clock. She checked everything, gave me a vaginal examination, and left around five o'clock, saying she would be back by seven. I was surprised she would come back so soon because according to stories I'd heard, cervical dilatation usually lasts much longer; however, knowing she would return shortly made me feel secure. At 6:30, I desperately wanted her to come back because I felt a strong urge to push. Ton encouraged me to stick it out until seven o'clock until Agaath came back.

Could you resist that urge?

I made an effort, but at a certain moment, I could no longer put up a fight. The funniest part was that Ton was so intensely involved in helping me puff and sigh that he got out of breath himself and couldn't go on. When he stopped sighing, I lost my motivation to continue and Florian could do as he liked.

Did you use the moment of complete cervical dilatation as an indicator to start pushing?

No. I didn't give the dilatation a minute's thought. I had drilled it into my head that I was not allowed to push because I would tear. So it was as if the baby was pushing and not me. From the moment the pushing contraction started, I sensed he wanted to get out.

Did you have contact with Florian during the delivery?

Yes, during the pushing contractions, I said to Ton, 'I bet it will be a little girl; our child is coming!'

Even when the head presented itself, I cried, 'how lovely, how lovely.'

TON: We ended up on the sofa. Mena had been hanging onto my neck during the contractions. She was quite willing to deliver standing in that position, but the floor was so slick I almost slipped so I put her on the sofa. I figured I could not hold Mena and catch the baby both. When the head become visible, I had an anxious moment. It is difficult when you really realize that a whole baby has to pass through such a narrow opening. When its little nose had come out, everything went so fast; the whole head was born after one pushing contraction.

That was a fantastic moment. Mena's vagina was so stretched by then that I was afraid she might tear. That is why I helped the upper and then the lower shoulder be born. After that, it was only a matter of putting my little fingers under the baby's armpits and pulling during another pushing contraction, before Florian was born. Thinking back, I am still amazed that it went so smoothly.

Do you feel that you did things the right way?

META: Because everything went so easily, it would have been hard to have done anything wrong.

At a certain point, you decided to sigh and puff rather than to begin pushing because you were afraid you might tear. Did your body know what to do instinctively?

META: I had not paid any attention to the breathing. That was Ton's job. I am convinced that everything would have been much more difficult if he hadn't done that. Without him, I would not have bothered. He started breathing and simply kept going even when I kept stopping because the urge to push was so strong that I could not continue. I could start up with him after the urge had subsided.

What did you do with the umbilical cord?

TON: Agaath handled that. We had just recovered from Florian's first cry when she rang the doorbell. She was rather surprised when I opened the door with a big grin on my face and said that she might as well leave the birthchair in her car. Nevertheless, I was relieved she had arrived.

MENA: Agaath helped me with the afterbirth. I did not know that I needed to push once more; Florian had arrived by himself so I thought the afterbirth would come of its own accord, too.

Did you feel a sense of recognition when you first saw Florian?

MENA: Florian was someone totally new, a character on his own, a totally new human being.

TON: I still don't have the feeling—except now and then—that it is our child, or my child. It feels as though we have a guest staying with us. In the beginning, I had a strange feeling that someone might come and take him away the next day.

META: This reaction is partly because the child is already so much an individual. Physically, he resembles both Ton and myself, of course; everyone who comes by debates which one of us he looks like.

Do you have a closer connection with Florian now that you have known him for two months?

MENA: Yes, we are getting closer. At the birth, he was still so far away.

TON: When he smiles at us, we think the relationship is forming. But is he smiling at us exclusively, or does his smile still have little to do with happiness and recognition?

What was the first bodily contact with Florian like?

MENA: Very weird. I could not believe it. Ton put him on my stomach immediately, all wet and naked. I said, 'It seems like Christmas.' Christmas is very special to me; you wait a long time, and, suddenly, you are very happy. Later, I told Ton that I could almost believe in the stork again: one moment, there is nothing; the next, a baby is lying on your stomach. Such a tiny creature, totally naked. Where has he come from? This feeling, especially powerful during the first few days, has stayed with me.

Vertical Delivery and First Contact:
A Midwife's Perspective

ONE OF THE most recent developments in your practice is to intervene as little as possible during the birth. How did this come about?

AGAATH: During my training at the School of Midwives, we only saw deliveries in which the woman was supine or half sitting. We were taught how to maneuver the baby's shoulders. The shoulders have to turn within the pelvis; this does not happen spontaneously in the supine position. We were taught to move the baby's head down slightly in the direction of the anus so the upper shoulder can pass along the pubic bone. Then you maneuver the head up toward the pubic bone so the lower shoulder can be born.

Once one has been in practice and witnessed countless deliveries, one discovers that such techniques are invariably unnecessary because of the force of the gravity when the mother is in the vertical position. The only task left is to help the child onto the pillow, which lies in front of the woman, as it is born. Your job is to ensure a soft landing.

Has your involvement with the vertical birth altered your attitude as a midwife?

I feel very strongly that I am only there in case I am really needed, and I hold back more and more. In my mind, it is important not to be in the limelight too much. My position as midwife should be a modest one; I am more or less a guest at the delivery, and it is very important for the people involved to do a lot together without the midwife. I am there to solve problems and to make sure all goes well. When everything progresses

smoothly, there is really no task for me. Then, I simply show faith in the successful outcome of the delivery and that, I believe, is the most important part of my work.

Is the delivery more pleasant for the woman if she is left to herself like that?

I think this is very important, particularly during a vertical delivery. I feel that letting the woman have a more natural delivery helps the connection between mother and child, and also between father and child. In the old days, the midwife or the doctor 'performed' the delivery, but nowadays a woman feels that she has done it herself: 'I have delivered a child, supported by my husband, a girlfriend…we have done it together.' It is a memorable experience, one that will be carried with them all their lives. We, however, wash our hands and disappear from their lives.

Does the idea of letting nature run its course influence your instructions during the pushing?

During my training, I learned that a woman had to hold up her legs, take a big breath, put her chin on her chest, and then push. In the vertical birth, however, it is obvious the expulsive force is vital, and the woman merely yields to that force and pushes with these waves. When she is in the second stage, and the head protrudes a little bit, we advise her to suppress the pushing urge as long as she can. When the urge becomes too strong, she can push a bit and breathe away the remaining part of the contractions. In this

position, many women know what to do instinctively.

What happens when the delivery is over and the child is born?

You may remember the old days—when a child was born it was briefly held up and shown to its mother, who was lying in her bed. Then it was taken away, bathed, clothed, and put in a cradle. Luckily, this no longer happens. After that, there was a period when the child was put on the mother's tummy immediately, although she could hardly see it since she was lying on her back. When we first started working with the vertical method, we gave the baby to its mother immediately. But then we decided not to pick it up for the mother, and we saw something totally different happen; namely, the woman first watches the child as it lays naked in front of her. She can look at it. 'Is it a boy or a girl?' is never asked. Mothers can see this for themselves and, at the same time, can check whether the child is intact and healthy.

Then they start to touch it, feeling the baby's hands, feet, and head, and, very often, they pick up the baby after several minutes have elapsed. Frequently, the women pick up their babies much later than the midwife would have done. A woman looks at and touches her baby much longer than I ever imagined. It is very special and beautiful to watch.

What happens then? Do you suck out the baby's mouth?

Nowadays, I suck a child's mouth

only when I see it is really needed. I don't when the baby looks fine. There are a number of reasons this sometimes has to be done. For instance, when the amniotic fluid contains meconium; when the child inhales this, it can settle in the lungs and cause problems. If the amniotic fluid is clear, however, the lungs can cope with it. The fluid will be resorbed and will not trouble the child.

Dr. Michel Odent advocates putting a baby on its side in the so-called safety position. But a child is born that way anyway, isn't it?

Children are usually born lying on their sides. The shoulders turn within the pelvis, so they come out this way naturally. This turns out to be the best position. Lying on its side, the baby can spit out the mucus and amniotic fluid spontaneously and let it dribble out its mouth. Positioning a child on its back would prevent this from happening.

Do you leave the child with its mother for a long time after the birth?

If possible, the baby stays with her for one hour; after that, I examine it, do routine tests, and dress it. Some tests are done immediately after the delivery but these take very little time. You can almost do these unnoticed. After an hour, I check to see if everything functions well: listen to the heartbeat and lungs and check the reflexes. I usually do this in a warm environment—on top of the mother's belly, for instance, as she is nice and warm lying in bed. When your hands are warm and you take your time, the child doesn't mind.

Would it mind less if you had done it fifteen minutes after the delivery?

When you do it that soon, babies of-ten start to scream and cry because they panic, not knowing where they are and what is happening to them. It was shocking to see this practice in a German film called *Natural Birth,* which showed hospital deliveries in Germany. Almost all the deliveries were artificial. After the babies were born, they were held up, shown to the mother, and taken swiftly to a separate room to be checked. From the crying, you could tell that the child was panic stricken and incredibly unhappy.

Later, when I caught myself checking the child too early, I heard that same cry. I knew that this was not right; I must handle it differently. Indeed, if you leave the baby alone with its mother a little longer, invariably, it will undergo all the procedures quietly without being seized by panic. I believe by that time it calms down and has had a chance to orient itself.

Sometimes a mother wants to put her baby to her breast to feed it immediately after the delivery. Is she often successful?

No. The baby absolutely is not ready for it then. After approximately fifteen to twenty minutes the baby usually is and indicates this very clearly by searching for the nipple and making sucking movements. The notion that a newborn baby cannot feel and is unable to do anything is absolutely wrong. The child shows us when it is or isn't enticed by something.

It is common practice to bathe the baby relatively soon after the birth. Do you do this?

As far as I am concerned, there is no need to bathe the baby. Babies used to be considered dirty at birth, so they were bathed. Babies do not enjoy a quick cleaning, though they love to relax in warm water. A mother may enjoy giving her baby a bath immediately after the deliv-ery. A midwife can put a washbowl next to the mother so she can bathe the baby. Of late, I encourage men to occupy themselves with this, partly because they are often quite reticent about doing something with their babies. They are scared of handling them too roughly or hurting them. Often, they fear this tiny human being. When you urge a father to bathe his child, many times you see how they enjoy fussing over the child. In this way, you can help establish their first contact. Later, many fathers say 'That was a beautiful moment.'

Women often talk to their babies. Do fathers do this as well?

Fathers seem to be more diffident in that respect. I believe they talk more when they are alone with their babies. A few times, I've been in another room and have overheard a father chatting away to his child. Perhaps men feel inhibited to talk baby talk or something like that.

What is the task of the maternity nurse?

She has a very important role. During the delivery, she assists the midwife; she organizes the household, prepares what is needed, and assists during the stitching. After the delivery, she takes care of mother and child. In consultation with the midwife, she offers advice about the baby's care. She assists the new mother by word and deed—counseling her and, maybe more important, keeping the household going, which is indispensable when there are other children.

She coordinates visitors so the mother can get enough rest. The excellent maternity aid system in the Netherlands is part of the reason we have such a low perinatal death rate, a reason that is often underestimated.

BY DR. G. J. KLOOSTERMAN

The Effect of the Midwife and Home Delivery on Modern Obstetrics

PRACTICALLY EVERYONE is intrigued with the phenomenon of pregnancy and birth. The most likely explanation for this universal interest is that through procreation people regard themselves as links in a human chain, extending from long before their own births until long after their deaths. In this way, individuals contribute to it a type of eternity. The ability to extend influence beyond one's life span may be one reason men have often compared creating art or making contributions to science to the birth process. Anthropologist Margaret Mead may have been closer to the truth than many people admit when she asserted that human societies, which have been defined almost exclusively by men, reflect male jealousy or women's capacity to give birth and thus to continue humanity directly. The battle over which gender is stronger is found everywhere in mythology and folk tales.

A consequence of male interest and curiosity surrounding pregnancy and delivery is the development of obstetrics and its tendency in many cultures to discount the role of midwives. A good obstetrician (traditionally male) and a good midwife (traditionally female) approach birth from markedly different perspectives. Obstetricians direct their attention toward detecting and treating pathological problems, whereas midwives take great pride in watching the course of a normal delivery in which the woman in labor maintains authority for the birth and does the work by herself. People can become meddlesome and overstep boundaries when a subject fascinates them. The desire to di-

rect the delivery, taking power for giving birth away from the woman and, thus, granting themselves the honor of bringing forth new life, can be very strong for obstetricians.

Many obstetric "advances" have presented certain drawbacks, and during some periods of history, the obstetrician was much more of a danger than a blessing for the woman in labor. At the end of the nineteenth century, the safest place to deliver was at home under a midwife's guidance. During this period, in some months 20 percent of young mothers died at the academic hospital in Vienna. In the mid-1800s, a Dr. Semmelweis observed that doctors transmitted bacteria to women during labor, which often resulted in their deaths. His discovery, one of the most important in the history of medicine, reveals the type of tragedy that can occur when obstetrics intervenes with a natural process. It is not my intention to belittle the achievements of obstetrics. The birth process is safer today than ever before for the woman who has a narrow pelvis or other obstacles to giving birth to a healthy child. Women with severe circulatory problems or whose baby is in a transverse position as well as those who give birth to twins or triplets benefit tremendously from the progress obstetrics has made. However, the great majority of all expectant women can conceive, carry the child, go into labor, and deliver without medical intervention. Obstetrics does benefit healthy women indirectly by giving them reassurance that if something does go wrong they have someplace to turn. A

major contribution of obstetrics is the practice of examining pregnant women regularly so many problems can be detected at any early stage. Perhaps more important, and often forgotten, is for the majority of women each checkup provides an opportunity to be told that everything is fine, and this emotional support has a positive effect.

As the field of obstetrics developed, the percentage of hospital deliveries increased. Scientific evidence to support hospitalization for routine deliveries does not exist. The reasons given for delivering in a hospital play on a woman's fear that something may go wrong and in the hospital she would be near medical personnel and equipment that could save her life or that of her child. In reality, most women do not gain anything from giving birth in a hospital.

Proponents of hospital births argue that a woman who wants a nautral birth can have one in a hospital as satisfactorily as at home, while at the same time having the security of knowing help is close at hand if needed. In most hospitals, this is far from the case, and even if everyone involved were to attempt to provide a woman with the birth experience she deserves, it is unlikely that a hospital delivery would be as fulfilling as a home delivery. The reason for this being that a hospital is no place for the unpredictable, and therefore no place for the individual. Medical staffs work in an orderly fashion, adhering to hierarchy and regulations, and expecting discipline and punctuality. Upon being admitted to a hospital, a woman enters an alien world where she cannot be herself to the extent she can be at home. When she brings her baby into the world in her own environment, the midwife (or obstetrician) is her guest and has to ask her where to find the diapers or the kitchen. The woman in labor is the one giving instructions. As soon as a woman steps into a hosptial, she must adapt to a foreign environment. Her independence is taken away from her. She must ask whether she may have something to eat (and will often be refused, especially in the United States, because her doctor may decide to perform a Cesarean section), she loses much say in whether she will be given medication, and she may have to ask permission to use the restroom—and then where to find it. Some hospitals still require the partner to remain in the waiting room, and objections from the couple about being separated fall on deaf ears. In many hospitals, a woman's pubic hair is shaved and she is given an enema regardless of how she feels about these procedures. If she resists, hospital rules and regulations are cited. She may be told that walking in the corridors during labor is not allowed. And some hospitals will require a woman to push in the supine position, her legs up in stirrups, which is the most unnatural birth position possible. Vertical delivery—using the birthchair or supported squatting position, which women will assume instinctively—is much more logical and, as has been confirmed by scientific research, increases the chance of a spontaneous delivery. In some countries, women are given episiotomies as a

matter of course. At one time in Germany, this practice caused a great deal of controversy because Turkish women living there ardently objected to the unnecessary procedure and were finally exempted from it, though all other first-time mothers continued to be given episiotomies. After a hospital delivery when a mother stretches out her arms to hold her newborn, she will often hear the following admonishment: "Do not touch the baby with your dirty hands." Her hands are considered dirty because the doctor and nurses are wearing sterile gloves and she is not. Yet her bacteria will be on the child very soon regardless, and furthermore, the child has already received antibodies through the placenta against the mother's bacteria. (In fact for this reason, the only person who is not "dirty" is the mother: doctors, nurses, and other hospital staff are truly dangerous for the newborn baby because they carry bacteria that often are resistant to antibiotics.) After the mother has seen her child briefly—sometimes already dressed and lying in a cradle—the baby is taken away to the nursery. Often, the mother can only have contact with her baby when she insists on breastfeeding, and then the infant will be brought to her for feeding, after which he or she is promptly returned to the nursery. When mothers complain, the policy is defended by the argument that this arrangement is more hygienic. But nurseries have been shown to be the most unhygienic measure conceivable. Mother and child belong with each other, and from a bacteriological as well as a psychological

point of view it is dangerous when this unity is broken after the birth. In the communal environment of a nursery, babies are exposed to bacteria from other babies, other nurses, and hospital staff.

The ideal hospital delivery would be one in which the hospital functions merely as a hotel for healthy women who can deliver a baby without medical intervention. Until the institutional nature of the hospital is challenged, a hospital will consider someone who is admitted and who occupies a bed as a patient. A pregnant woman is labeled a patient, though she is in the final stages of a natural process having nothing to do with deterioration of health. To call her a patient is wrong, but even more objectionable is that she is treated as a patient as well.

Women should feel free to walk around and do as they please to make themselves more comfortable during labor. But because of the patients who are in a hospital because they are sick—as opposed to healthy expectant mothers, it is infeasible to allow women this freedom or to bend regulations to accommodate their partners during or following the birth, such as allowing them into the hospital in the middle of the night because they are just dying to see the baby. Desires that would not seem out of the ordinary or extravagant at a home birth are viewed by hospitals as problems. This lack of willingness to acknowledge and to try to fulfill a woman's individual needs can erode her self-confidence, sense of independence, and self-respect. In this unaccepting foreign environment, her state of mind will be far from the positive state that characterizes delivery in domestic surroundings.

Loss of emotional well-being is only one aspect of the negative impact of hospital deliveries for women anticipating routine deliveries. Hospitalization actually poses health risks to healthy expectant women because of increased intervention. One may think this is true for a small number of women only, certainly not for many, but that is not the case. In Sweden, the United States, Canada, West Germany, and England, where routine deliveries take place in hospitals, the percentage of medically intervened deliveries rises every year. The rate of some degree of intervention in these countries is four to five times as high as in Holland, where more than a third of all women deliver at home. In Canada and the United States, over 20 percent of babies are delivered by Cesarean section. And that is the national average. I visited a hospital in Canada where 30 percent of deliveries were Cesareans. When birthing in hospitals is compulsory, obstetricians and hospitals tighten the rules they've created and begin to treat problem and routine rights similarly because there is no danger that "business" will be low. If a culture, supported by the government and the medical profession, offers the choice of giving birth at home, hospitals will be forced to create a birthing environment that is more domestic and will allow births to progress naturally. Only by maintaining or returning to the tradition of home deliveries attended by midwives will obstetricians be prevented from monopolizing deliveries, and therefore regulating methods of giving birth to suit their needs rather than those of the women they're serving. The option of home delivery forces hospitals to adapt as much as possible within an institutional setting to the public's justified desires for a birth experience in which a woman who chooses to deliver there is considered capable of and given the freedom to direct the course of her delivery.

For women's physical and emotional well-being, the option of home delivery and the availability of midwives are important issues now more than ever. Obstetrics needs both obstetricians, who care for pregnant women with medical problems or whose deliveries truly require intervention, and midwives, who support women, the majority, who only need coaching. When obstetricians and hospitals monopolize obstetric care, and the important counterpart, the midwife, no longer exists or is made subservient to the doctor, women lose much say regarding a major event in their lives.

PART II

Influence of Water

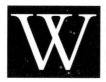HEN A WOMAN is in labor, her need for warmth is great. This explains the return to the tradition of using room temperature water during cervical dilatation. Almost all the women interviewed for this book felt that having a shower or bath helped them handle their contractions better.

Since 1977, the French obstetrician Michel Odent has pioneered the use of warm water baths instead of drugs to relieve pain and to relax women whose labors are long and/or difficult. The maternity ward at the hospital in Pithiviers, France, which he restructured using this approach, has had a high spontaneous birth rate. His experiences with labor and delivery in water have influenced obstetrics throughout the world.

The underwater delivery is still surrounded by controversy. For instance, the misconceptions that a child will suffocate before it surfaces or that a woman can get uterine or perineal infection by sitting in nonsterile water are still used as arguments against giving birth in water. A newborn cannot drown during the journey to the water's surface as long as he or she is attached to the mother by the umbilical cord. The child will not breathe until he or she is above water. Filling the tub adequately is essential to prevent any chance of the infant rising above the surface during the birth and taking water into the lungs through the nose or mouth. Odent has not encountered complications with the child's safety. Igor Tjarkovsky, a Russian biologist, researched underwater deliveries extensively, particularly the concern regarding infection. In his research of three hundred such deliveries, he didn't come across one case of infection, and he concludes there is no reason to assume that underwater birth causes infection.

Assisting at an Underwater Birth

TANJA GAVE BIRTH TO HER SECOND CHILD AT HOME IN A LARGE BATH IN HER SAUNA. THE FIRST TIME SHE DELIVERED IN BED. THE ADVANTAGE OF TANJA'S HUGE TUB IS THAT SHE HAD LOTS OF ROOM TO MOVE ABOUT, AND AMPLE SPACE ALLOWED HER HUSBAND TO JOIN HER IN THE BATH. THEY COULD SIT TOGETHER AND RETAIN THEIR INTIMACY. A NORMAL TUB PROVIDES ROOM FOR THE WOMAN ONLY, AND HER PARTNER SITS OR STANDS NEXT TO IT.

Did Tanja sit in the bath the whole time?

AGAATH: During the first part of the cervical dilatation, Tanja was upstairs in the living room. She sat on the sofa or walked around, hanging onto objects for support. But during the final part, as the contractions became more and more painful, she got into the bath.

What are the advantages of delivering in water?

It isn't beneficial so much during the delivery itself, but during the period prior to it, the dilatation, it has an extremely relaxing effect. The body can move around freely when not restrained by a chair, sofa, or bed. You feel much freer and your body becomes partially weightless. During the contractions, especially, you appreciate how lovely it is to relax, to let your body hang loose. Warm water is extremely relaxing, which makes you less aware of the pain.

The contractions increase in intensity because you are so relaxed, yet you don't experience stronger pain.

The delivery progresses faster. And the child loves to be in the bath with its mother after the delivery.

Would it be possible to step into a bath with your child after you have delivered vertically?

Yes, you could do that. If you step into a bath immediately after the delivery, the chances of uterine or perineal infection are small because, at that point, the pressure in the womb is still so high and there is still much contraction activity. If you got into a tub a few days after the delivery, the danger of infection would be greater.

Did Tanja change her position while she was in the bath?

At first, she was hanging forward over the edge to have the contractions, but when the pushing contractions start, it is often more comfortable to sit, leaning slightly backward.

Is there a gradual transition from the dilatation to the pushing contractions?

Yes, in general it is a rather gradual process, but sometimes the transition is quite abrupt. During the stronger contractions, a woman wants to push, which is not so much the case during the milder contractions. This urge to push gets stronger and stronger.

Is one allowed to push then?

Practically always. Often you hear women ask, 'I've got the urge to push, may I push now?' When women feel these pushing contractions, the cervical dilatation is almost always complete.

Did Tanja apply certain techniques to cope with the contractions?

Tanja does this in her own way. She didn't attend a pregnancy course as she didn't think that was necessary. She said 'I'll wait and see and deliver and breathe in my own way.' That was her attitude during both her deliveries. Basically, it is not necessary to attend a course to learn how to breathe. When you are in tune with you body and aware of your emotions, you can do it without breathing exercises. You discover for yourself how to breath, developing your own technique that suits you.

You held Tanja's hand and touched her belly. Why did you do that?

To be part of it, to simply support the woman in labor. It is a gesture that says I want to help her, even though I can't really do anything and she is the one suffering the pain. I often notice that women enjoy their bodies to be touched and caressed.

Did you have a good view of her perineum as she was sitting in the water?

With my hand, I could judge how far the head had descended, even though I couldn't see very well. Her bulging perineum told me that the baby would be born after a couple of contractions. Having a good view during this delivery wasn't as important as it usually is because Tanja had no perineal tears during her first delivery.

In a normal bathtub, however, you have a good view. The delivery should take place very slowly. I had planned to

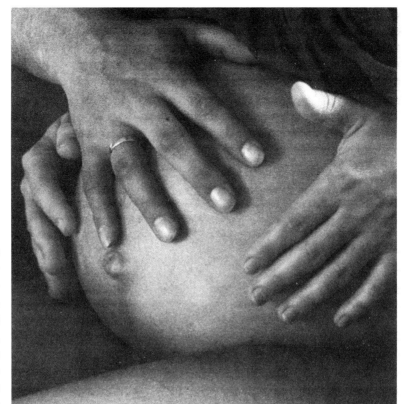

do Tanja's that way, but because it was my first underwater delivery, everything went very abruptly. I fished the baby out of the water immediately, in fact, perhaps too soon. The next time I shall do it differently; I'll let the baby be born more gently, let it float for a while before bringing it to the surface.

Many people wonder whether a baby who is born underwater will suffocate.

Several factors play a role in the child's breathing. First there is the discrepancy between the pressure of the womb and that of air. In this sense, the underwater delivery is advantageous because the transition from one pressure level to another is much smoother. The difference in temperature has a stimulating effect as well; when the baby moves from the warm, wet uterus into the colder air, it starts to breath. Shortage of oxygen is a third stimulus. The placenta stops functioning shortly after the birth, and, consequently, the decrease in oxygen supply results in an accumulation of carbon dioxide (CO_2) in the blood, which promotes breathing.

If a child is born quietly underwater, the breathing mechanism will not be triggered for a while because there is not the stimulus of coldness, of pressure difference, or an excessive level of CO_2. It is safe to let the baby be born without haste, after which it can come above the water.

Only then will the baby start to make breathing movements and the lungs unfold themselves.

How warm should the water be?

It is important for a child to be born in a warm environment, so the temperature of the bath in which Tanja's baby was born was about body temperature, 98.6 degrees, which is the temperature the baby was used to. Babies don't feel comfortable in the cold, and their body temperatures drop very quickly. When you bathe a baby right after the delivery, make sure the water is about body temperature so the baby can make the transition from life within the womb to one outside of it slowly.

You congratulated Tanja only after the placenta had been delivered. Is that customary practice?

Yes, to a midwife the delivery has come to a good end after the placenta has been born successfully. If everything is fine for both mother and child, the delivery is over and worth a few cheers.

The baby seemed so bright and awake after the birth.

Yes, it was obvious Jody sought con-

tact with her mother. The child needs to be a certain distance from the mother to actually see her. For both mother and child this is done most easily in the vertical position. She can hold and look at the baby at the same time. When the mother is lying down she has trouble seeing her child.

After the delivery, Tanja and her baby stayed in the water for forty-five minutes. Both of them thoroughly enjoyed it. The child was fully awake all that time. She looked around with bright eyes and sucked her mother's breast firmly. It must be delightful for the baby to come from a warm spot and go into another and to be totally free to move, not confined by towels or clothes.

Did Jody also look at you?

Yes, a baby is sensitive to soft sounds, and I think that is what caught her attention. At one point, I talked to her. I believe that if you allow a child to recover from the delivery for awhile and then deal with it in a gentle way the baby will be inclined to seek contact with you.

Was the baby disturbed by anyone while she played in the water with her mother for three-quarters of an hour?

With the exception of my cutting the umbilical cord, which was a little disruptive, no one touched the baby until Tanja indicated that she wanted to leave the bath.

Did the baby seem upset when you cut the cord?

We usually cut the umbilical cord about ten minutes after the baby's birth. This is about the time that the woman feels some afterpains, and the uterus contracts as a sign that the placenta is about to be born. You can see that the baby reacts to the cord being cut not because it hurts, but because foreign hands are touching its body. The baby, momentarily removed from its mother and made to alter its position, reacts apprehensively: 'What is happening now?' It is a disruption of the contact between mother and child.

On the one hand, you could delay cutting the cord, but if you were to cut it after the placenta was born the result would be a bit of a blood bath. That is why we do it after ten minutes. Often, the new father is asked to cut the cord as a symbolic gesture.

When you have to do something to the baby after one hour, it usually looks around quietly, whereas when you remove a child from its mother after only a quarter of an hour, the baby panics and screams and shouts for its mother. This hardly ever happens when you leave them together for an hour. Apparently, babies get used to the new situation by then.

Tanja felt very fit after the delivery, didn't she?

Almost all women who deliver in a vertical position—squatting, sitting, or standing—really enjoy remaining seated for awhile after the delivery, watching and holding their child. Afterwards, they get up by themselves, walk to the shower on their own accord, shower, and crawl into a clean bed. Almost all women can get up and walk after the delivery. Many women think that you can't muster the strength to do that, that you are weak right after the delivery. The reverse is true! Right after the delivery you feel very energetic and full of beans and are quite able to shower and walk around. When Tanja got out of the tub, she dried herself with a towel, got dressed, and went upstairs. She sat on the sofa with her older daughter and her baby for hours.

TANJA

Tanja: Jody's mother
Jody: second child, a girl (born at home)
Danny: first child, two-and-a-half-year-old-girl (born at home)
Michel: Jody's father
Agaath: midwife

THIS INTERVIEW TOOK PLACE TWO MONTHS AFTER JODY'S BIRTH.

You were the first woman in the Netherlands to deliver underwater. Had you told people of your plans?

TANJA: Just my family.

How did your family react?

They didn't quite approve of it. My sister-in-law asked a lot of questions since she might like to give birth this way, too. With her, I discussed breathing and that I had heard the baby sometimes swallows amniotic fluid.

I asked whether the baby could swallow the bath water. I also asked at what point they know whether the umbilical cord is wrapped round the head, because it is hard to see underwater. I didn't think about the rest.

Weren't you scared to be the first?

It was an experiment for me. I think it quite logical, anyway, to have the contractions underwater. Had they wanted to find out how long a child can stay underwater without breathing, like they seem to do in the United States, I wouldn't have done it. I don't see the point of that. Apparently, a baby is able to stay underwater for eighteen minutes.

With my first baby, my back ached terribly. During my pregnancy it already hurt, and when I had to push sitting in bed or lying on my side, it was too painful. I thought it logical to go into warm water. This time my back did not ache. I floated in the water; there was nothing to carry. When you are lying in bed and they put your legs up, it causes pressure on your tailbone.

The first time you delivered in bed?

Yes, in bed on my back. I laid in my bed the whole time. I painted my nails and had a pretty T-shirt on.

The second time, I got scared again when the contractions began. I eventually got out of bed and walked around downstairs. I should have gotten up at once and not have been so stupid as to try to stay in bed. You just don't know where to go. One is not mobile at all. In water it is not a problem.

Did you stay in the water the whole time?

From half past six until after eight o'clock. When Agaath arrived at half past four, I already was dilatated five centimeters.

How did you cope with the contractions before you got into the water?

By walking around and clinging onto the cupboard.

How did you decide to deliver in water? Of course, having a sauna you had an ideal bath.

My midwife gave me the idea. She said, 'If you wish, you can go into the big bath when the contractions start coming and even have your child there.' We actually didn't talk about it any more. I had watched a show about underwater deliveries on television.

Did that show convince you?

No, I didn't like the program. It was a Russian documentary with all these cats in water. I thought it was so sad. To me, that film was rather frightening because they kept the babies underwater. One child was even breastfed underwater, which gave me the creeps.

Michel went into the water with you. How did he feel about your desire to deliver there?

He agreed. He had a few questions like, 'What will they do if it starts breathing?' and 'What will they do if the child is not in the right position?' In the latter case, I would have had to go to the hospital anyway.

Did you find it embarrassing to be filmed?

No. If it had been my first child, I wouldn't have agreed to it. This time I knew I wouldn't be aware of the camera at all because with Danny I found that I didn't pay attention to who was coming or going. It was as if I were numbed. I have a very particular look on my face. You can see that on the film. Michel feels differently because he was not in a numbed state and was aware of being filmed.

A lot of people were there, too. Did that bother you?

No, I wanted them all to be there.

Were there many people at the first delivery?

My mother, my two sisters, the nurse, the midwife, and Michel.

Did you enjoy your mother's presence?

Yes, I held on to her tightly. I didn't let go of her. With Danny, when I delivered in bed, I held on to her hair, and all of them were obliged to pant, too. For hours on end. It lasted twenty-three hours. In the end, you just don't know where you are anymore, whether you are coming or going.

How long did the dilatation last this time?

About four to four and a half hours. Within two or three pushing contractions, she was here.

At that moment you were frightened. You said, 'I'm all on fire.'

I was scared because she came just like that. You often hear women say that the moment they think they will go mad the child is born.

This time you didn't pant much. Why?

The first time I really thought I was going to die. If you panic, you forget what happens to you and you can't enjoy it. When you get into a panic you tense up so all of you hurts even more.

This time you were not afraid?

This time I knew I wasn't going to die. I also didn't want to get into a panic because it frightens the others. That first time, my mother was so scared. She wanted me to go to hospital the entire time. Of course, it wouldn't have changed anything. Michel told me he thought I'd never be the same again, I looked so funny. I was so pathetic I was scared to death it would never come out. I remember think-ing, 'Nobody can have had so much pain. There isn't a soul in the world who can bear so much pain.' And because you are so tired, the push contractions don't come. In the end, I had no push contractions at all and had to push to Agaath's order. But that isn't the right way. It lasted so long. After Danny, I felt as if I had been in a car accident. I ached all over. My legs, my head, my arms, my neck. It really was abnormal. Veins in my nose had even burst.

After the second delivery, I had no pain at all. I got up and dressed. Of course, that's because I hadn't been lying with my legs in the air and my chin against my chest. This time, the pushing contractions came on very easily because I wasn't so exhausted. I'm inclined to think that even if you refrain from pushing, the child will come out on its own accord. This time, in the end, it rather frightened me because I couldn't hold back. I felt like keeping my legs together. I thought perhaps I could hold on to it a little longer. When you have got that feeling, you cooperate.

When the baby and placenta had been delivered, I really wanted to leave the bath right away. I no longer enjoyed the water. But when we started to play with her, it was really comfortable again. I thought 'The water may be slightly dirty, but what difference does it make?'

The afterbirth is foul. I think Agaath and Beatrijs think it is beautiful. I regard it as an organ, like a liver.

What did you do with the placenta?

I buried it after five days. It had been in the corridor, but we had forgotten all about it. I wouldn't dream of making broth from it as some people do.

What does it feel like when the placenta is delivered? Do you have to push or does it come one its own?

You push a little bit. You feel that something has to come out. It means that the end of the delivery is in sight, which is rewarding. You get a few contractions, and with the second child you get after-pains.

You didn't have those with your first child?

Not with the delivery of the placenta, although I did during breastfeeding. The pains are beneficial, of course, because that is how the womb reassumes its normal proportions. The afterpains I had with the second child are similar to the contractions that begin delivery. It is just as if the delivery starts all over. The afterpains lasted an afternoon. With my first child, I didn't experience the birth of the placenta, because I was unconscious. When she showed it to me afterwards, I was scared to death.

What was it like to have Jody on your belly immediately after she was born?

Fantastic. For Michel and me that was the most precious moment. The way they used to take away the baby immediately was horrendous. Danny was also put on my belly right away.

What was Jody's birth like for Michel? Was he afraid it wouldn't go well?

No, he was resolved not to be afraid again because he knew it would hurt and

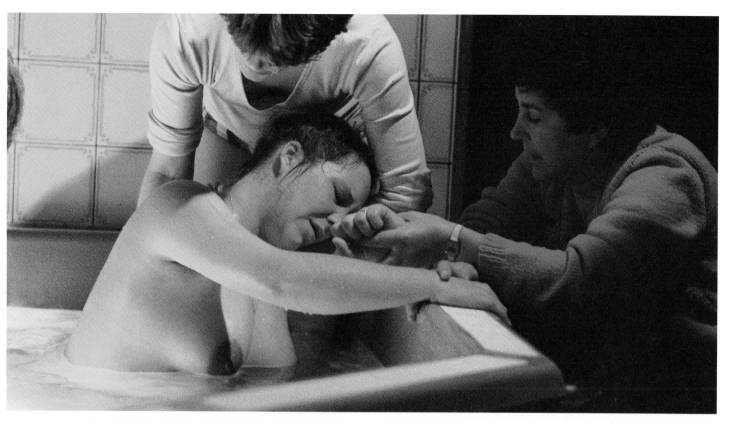

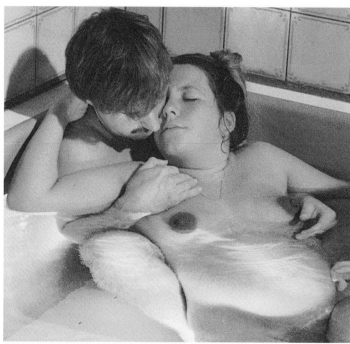

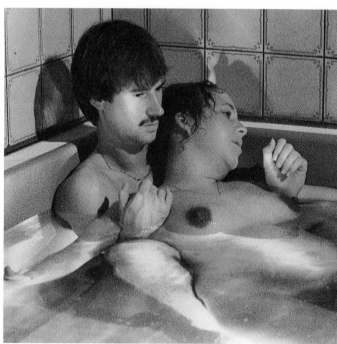

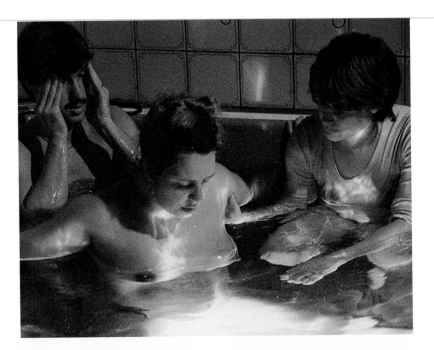

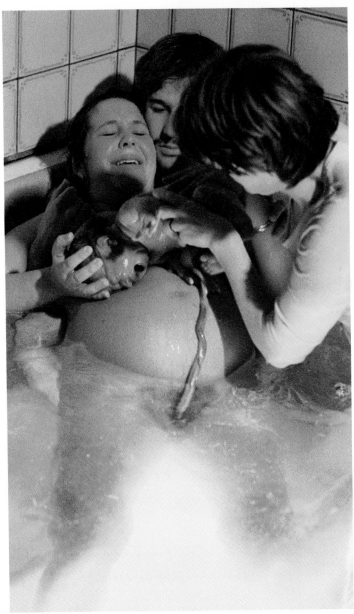

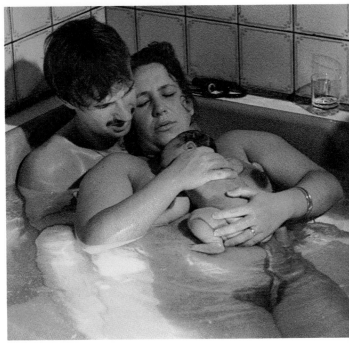

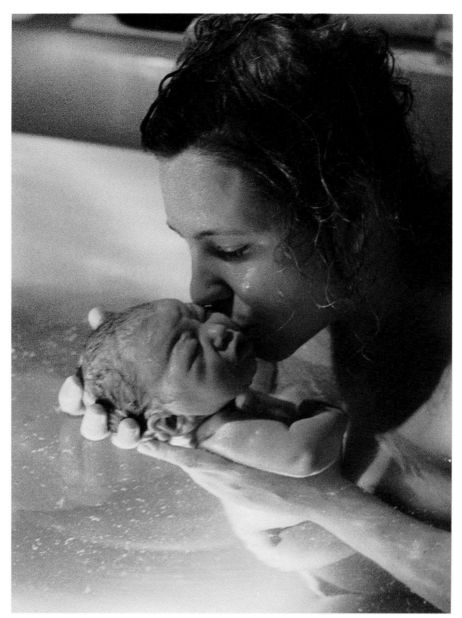

knew he couldn't do anything about it. The only thing he could do was massage my back and be with me. He behaved quite differently this time. Last time, he was very quiet and looked sort of greenish. It made him sick. This time, he saw the child coming very slowly, and he found that more exciting.

During your pregnancy, were you very conscious of the child within you? Did you feel that you knew it already? Did you give it a name?

Names caused me nightmares. I postponed coming up with them as long as possible. I hadn't even thought about it. Actually, only the evening she had arrived, did we think of a name. At the hair salon

that I own, I talked with every client about their deliveries or about their children. There wasn't a pregnant woman who came in that I did not keep talking in her chair for hours.

I can't think of anything better than reading about childbearing and looking at photographs. I keep a diary every week.

With the first child, feeling movement inside of me was so wonderful. The second time, too, I was constantly aware of having somebody within me. It was so cozy. When I was alone, I had the feeling that there were two of us. On our skiing holiday, at which time I was five months pregnant, I wasn't allowed to ski too much. When the others went out skiing, I felt I wasn't alone. Often, I had the feeling,

'I'm the lucky one to have a child in my womb!' I looked awful at parties for I wore one of those impossible dresses, but I didn't care two hoots. I'm very aware of the fact that men can never experience anything like this. Michel found Danny's birth to be the most exciting thing he had ever experience, although beforehand he had rather dreaded the moment. Afterwards, he said, 'It was the most beautiful thing I've ever seen.' Even now. It didn't interest him much to feel the baby moving before she was born. When the contractions started, he got frightfully nervous. Normally, he isn't a nervous person. I felt privileged.

Is the time shortly before the birth and the

birth itself the best period of the whole preg-nancy?

Yes. About three weeks before the baby is due, you start thinking about it very much because you think it may come at any moment.

When I was only just pregnant with Jody, I started rereading all the books I had read when I was pregnant with Danny and looked at all the photographs of a baby during pregnancy. Sometimes I got scared when I thought 'If something goes wrong now, it will never be right.' For instance, the lungs develop during such and such a week. Then I'd think, 'What do I have to do in order for all to go well?' I was very frightened something might go wrong.

Were there many things you had to take into account when you were pregnant? Did your pregnancy incapacitate you in any way?

I had to be careful about smoking and also about lifting because it puts pressure on your womb. I didn't jump down the stairs, and I took care not to bump into things. Otherwise, I did everything I normally do.

When Jody was born you climbed the stairs at once and walked down with Danny in your arms.

My two births were so different. I couldn't think of leaving my bed with Danny; I felt dead. Not so with Jody. I sat on the couch until twelve o'clock. Only then did I feel sleepy.

With Danny, I perspired like anything the moment I left the bed. When I got up, the perspiration ran down my chin. It was July. I couldn't even make coffee.

This time I perspired, too, but only at night. I can smell when I am ill. It's a completely different odor. That's how I know I am weak. When I go to the sauna I perspire like crazy, but it doesn't smell. After a birth, it's like having a fever. With Jody it didn't last more than three weeks, but with Danny it lasted at least three months.

I felt very depressed after Danny. Now, I am rather depressed, too. I'm suspicious about everything, but with Danny I made much more fuss. One morning I woke up and it was gone. I have had clients who told me that they were admitted to the hospital for postpartum depression. Perhaps I don't feel so bad this time because I knew the depression would come. Fortunately, doctors pay more attention to the problem now.

With Danny, I was very ill-tempered during my pregnancy. I threw everybody out of my house. People weren't allowed to say, 'You should drink milk.' I would get furious. I wanted Danny to have brown eyes, and when somebody said they were green, I had a fit. Some people asked, 'Are you sick?' 'No, I am not sick,' I'd tell them. 'Then the baby will be born bald, for the baby's hair rubs against the stomach wall and that's what makes you sick.' Well, if that were true, I would have vomited every day because she was born with long hair. Now, I don't listen. When people say, 'Let her cry. It's good for the lungs,' I say, 'Yes, indeed, excellent for the lungs,' and I comfort Jody. Isn't that what

I am here for? Then she is quiet. I think she has the right to cry if she wants to be with us, but I don't let her continue to cry. I just go and get her.

You went back to work quite soon after Jody's birth, didn't you?

After two weeks. With Danny, I went back to work two and a half weeks after the birth, which was too soon. I had decided that if I felt as weak as I did with Danny, I wouldn't go back to work for five or six weeks. But I did not.

Many women complain that breastfeeding restricts their freedom, that they can no longer work, and that the child ties them down too much.

I have never bothered weighing the baby after meals or questioned whether I could breastfeed. It is nonsense to think about these things. When your milk production falls, you have to be persistent and it will come back, at least that's what I've read. In the beginning, the maternity nurse weighed my babies, but as soon as she left, I returned the scales. Besides, I don't understand how the whole thing works. Every time I weighed her she weighed 6.6 pounds! I don't feed her with my right breast just because she had her last meal on the left one; I give her the breast that is bothering me most or give her both of them. I will take Jody to work with me until I stop breastfeeding her. I have an assistant who manages the business when I am not available. I also have a cleaning lady. I work from nine to six o'clock every day, except Fridays when

I work from one to eleven o'clock. She sleeps in the daytime and at night she wants to be with me, which is very pleasant, as if she knows that I have time for her then. Danny did the same thing.

As if they adapted to your rhythm?

Business comes first when you are your own boss. One solution would be to share child-care duties with your husband. That is a lovely idea; however, few companies would cooperate. In Sweden, the situation for young parents is much more favorable. The woman gets a six-month maternity leave, and the husband can stay at home for six months, too. The idea that a man takes off work to be with his baby is unheard of here in Holland.

How long did you breastfeed Danny?

I breastfed Danny for seven and a half months, after that I was fed up. My clothes were always dirty. Toward the end, I breastfed her in the morning and evening only and supplemented with porridge and vegetables. The less you feed your baby, the less milk you produce. I heard of someone whose doctor asked her how old her baby was and if she was still breastfeeding. After she answered, he said, 'This isn't the jungle you know.' I think I would have killed the guy. At a certain point, they start eating what you are eating and then breastfeeding stops naturally. In the beginning, when someone even mentioned Jody, the milk would start flowing. When I wear a wide dress, the milk runs down my legs to the ground. When she cries, the milk flows in every possible direction. I know when Michel and I make love, I'll almost float out of bed.

Breastfeeding takes a lot of time. Is this a problem for Michel?

Michel thinks breastfeeding is best. If she was bottle-fed, everyone would want to feed her, and Michel doesn't think that is good for the baby. As long as the baby is happy and content, that's what is important, all the rest can wait for awhile.

I don't think I would have any sympathy for jealousy about breastfeeding. Breastfeeding prevents you from return-

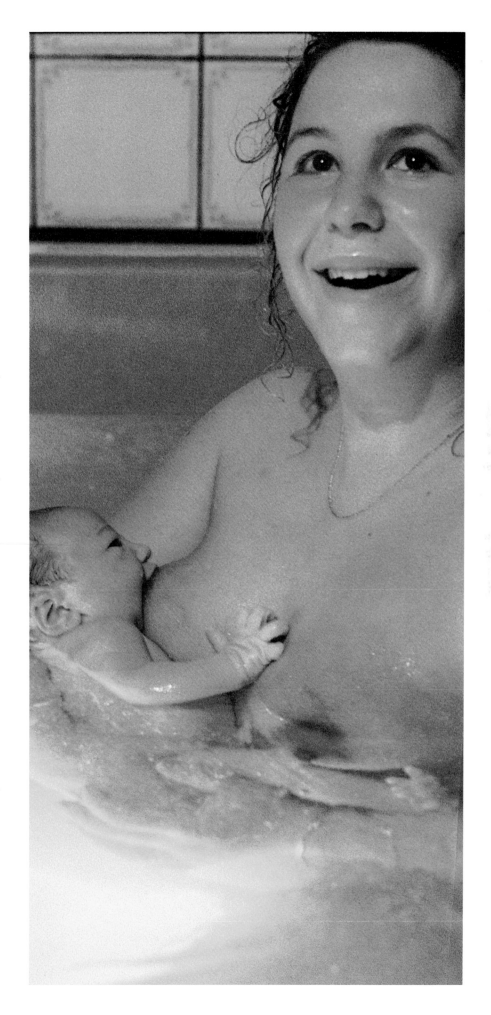

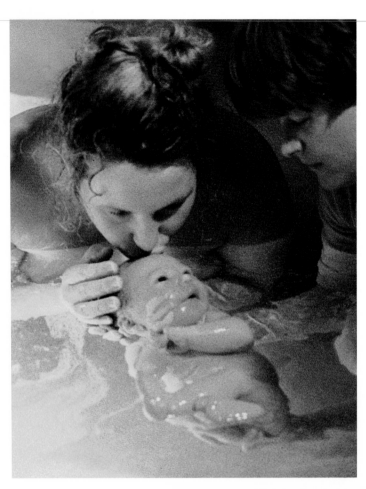

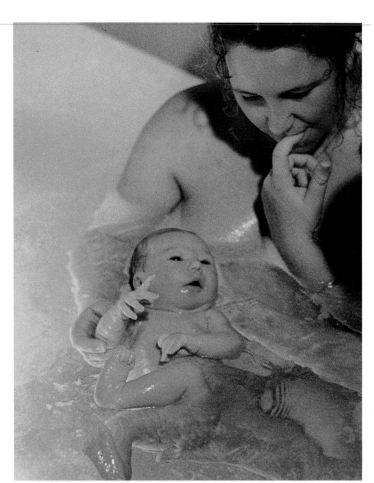

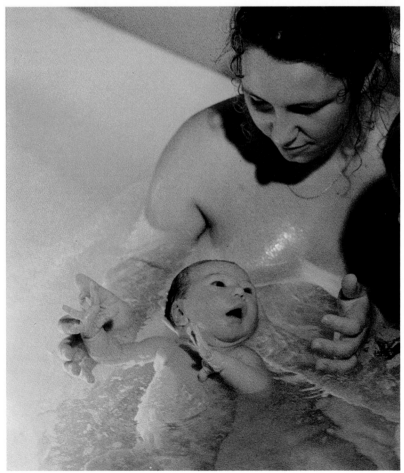

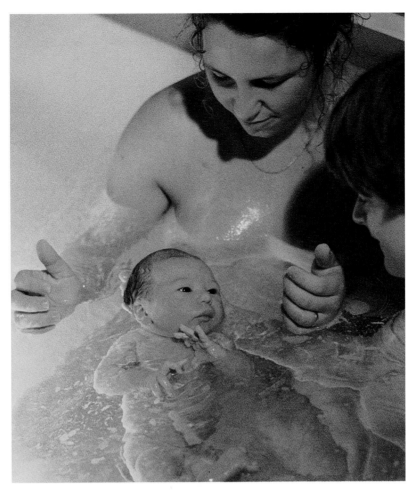

ing to hormonal equilibrium. This manifests itself in your sex life. He'd better forget that for awhile because I just don't feel like it. I don't have the patience for sex right now, especially since she sleeps in our room with us. I rush out of bed at the slightest sound to look at her, so he had better just go to sleep. Late at night, I usually breastfeed her in bed when he is sound asleep next to us. I hear him complain from time to time, but I don't attach much importance to it, knowing that all will be well in the end.

Jody sleeps in your bedroom. Many people think a child should have its own room.

I feel that you shouldn't always analyze things too much but should do what makes you feel most comfortable. Even if we had ten rooms, she'd still sleep with me. As a baby, Danny always slept with us. I could put the cradle in Danny's room, but then Jody would wake Danny.

In the last two weeks, Jody has slept in the cradle for about five hours and spent the rest of the night in bed with me. I never roll on top of her. After all, I never roll onto Michel either. I always put my arm around her and make sure the blanket doesn't cover her face. Besides, she'll start struggling if the blanket is over her head. Some nights she lies on top of me for hours. When I wake up in the morning, my arm has gone to sleep and every part of my body aches, but she has slept wonderfully. She simply snores away on top of me. Nowadays, Danny never sleeps with us. She always used to. I am not such a firm believer in letting older children sleep with their parents.

I explained to Danny that I couldn't sleep well with her because she kicked in her sleep. She understand and has not asked to sleep in bed with me again. When I was pregnant, I told her there simply wasn't space due to my big belly, and she accepted that immediately.

How has Danny reacted to Jody?

Really well. Now she is very sweet to Jody. She behaved badly the first week. She turned her volume up to ten and stamped her feet and battered the baby on the head, which was frightening. She wanted to get at me. When I was breastfeeding the baby, she would do something so I had to get up, but this passed in about a week. Once, about four weeks ago, she bit Jody's finger. Jody started to scream, and I slapped Danny's cheek. Jody had a blue finger, and Danny had a red cheek. I asked her, 'Why do you bite her?' 'She is naughty.' But now she is wild about her.

Did you ever talk about the delivery with Danny?

Four weeks ago she was sitting on the bed with me and asked whether the baby had come out my navel. 'But where did she come from then?' 'Here.' 'With blood? Did it hurt?' She often has pain defecating, so I said, 'It hurt exactly like that.'

It was then that we showed her the film of the birth—most of it without the sound. She thought it strange that Michel

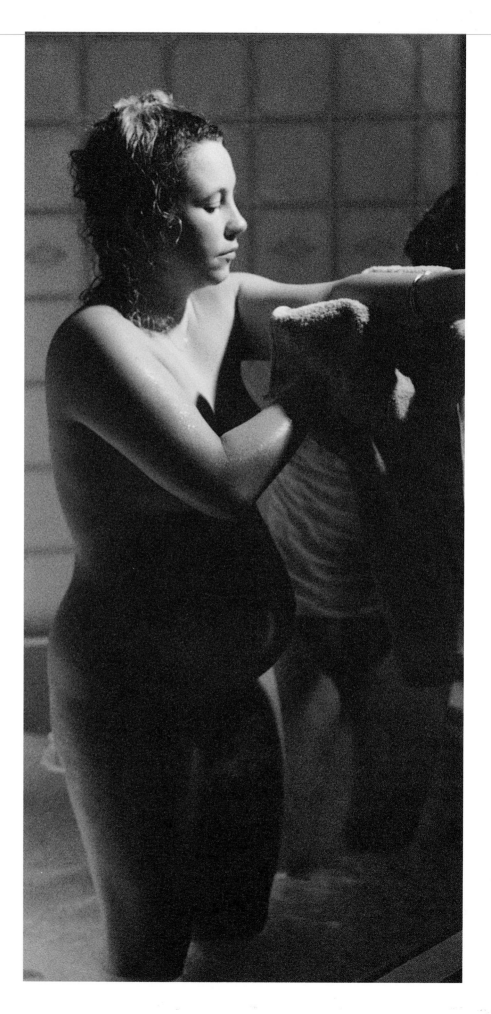

had been there. She kept asking, 'What is Papa doing now?' I answered, 'Nothing, he is only sitting in the water with me.' When Jody came out, she was thrilled, and we switched on the sound so she could hear Jody cry and us talk. After that, I skipped parts of the video until she was in it too. She thought the delivery was very weird. Now she asks me over and over whether there is another Jody in my belly.

Do you feel Jody reacts to your voice?

I am convinced she does. She is familiar with my voice because she hears me talk all day. I am sure she must get tired of it in the end. Presumably, she also knows Michel's voice and those of people who are around often.

In the beginning, when I was breast-feeding her, she sat very close to me and could focus well. I was the first thing she really saw clearly. If she had been given to another woman right after the delivery, she would have loved her, too, although I think it helps that she was familiar with my voice and my movements. When I walk around with her, she becomes quiet; Michel does not have the same effect on her. She is always making sounds, chatting with him. With me, she is always silent. When she was unhappy in the beginning, I would put her in the sling and go out walking or keep her close to me while I cooked.

She also knows my smell. She seems to sniff away all day long. I don't use perfume and certainly wouldn't put on any now. She goes into the bath and the shower with me. She doesn't mind getting her face wet. She loved being naked with me. She holds on to me with her arms and with her feet. When I kiss her feet, her toes grab my nose. She is just like a little ape, feeling with her hands and feet.

The first time I took Danny into the sauna, she was three months old. I could tell when she had had enough. Then we'd go into the Turkish bath, not into the cold water of course.

Was Jody awake much in the days following the delivery?

She was awake for a considerably long time after the delivery, almost four hours. It was a great joy to watch Jody swim like that. She cried for a moment, but she let herself be hushed at once. Danny, on the other hand, fell asleep immediately, but her delivery had been much tougher. Jody was and is often awake, looking around a lot of the time. She smiled after one week, whereas Danny's smile didn't appear until the fifth week.

Is the second child easier because you are more experienced as a mother?

Yes, you are more relaxed. You don't panic so quickly. Before I had Danny, I had never touched a baby in my life because I wasn't fond of them. I felt apprehensive about holding someone else's baby. With Danny, when bathing her slippery body for instance, I felt awkward, because everything was new to me.

You wonder whether you are doing things the way they are supposed to be done. You have to build up some self-confidence and not listen to other people's endless advice. When you let others influence you too much, you only get more confused because everyone has a different opinion.

Are you more secure now?

Yes, of course. Now the novelty is having two children. On the other hand, I carry Jody more naturally and am more relaxed about everything. From her cries, I can tell what is the matter. I have always been able to do that with her. One night I couldn't fall asleep, though she was sound asleep. Out of the blue, she vomited. Michel sees that as proof of my maternal instincts. I was simply waiting for something to happen. Afterwards, I could go to sleep. Intuition is built into you, and as long as you trust in that, everything goes somewhat better.

PAMELA AND FRANS

Pamela: Roland's mother
Roland: first child, a boy (born at home)
Frans: Roland's father
Beatrijs: midwife

THIS INTERVIEW TOOK PLACE FOUR AND A HALF MONTHS AFTER ROLAND'S BIRTH.

You constructed a bath. Did you do that with the intention of delivering in it or only to relax in during cervical dilatation?

PAMELA: I was well informed about the possibility of delivering in a bath, but my intention was to use it only to have my contractions. I had read about Michael Odent, the French obstetrician, who advises everyone delivering at home to get into the bath. The idea appealed to me.

FRANS: Our midwife told us about a shop that sold plastic tubs. The price wasn't too bad, so we bought one. Pamela got into it with her big belly, and we found that the greater part of her body was still above water. So I bought a second, identical tub and joined the two together.

How did you keep the water temperature high enough?

FRANS: We filled the tub and regulated its temperature by adding more warm water when the tub cooled down.

PAMELA: I sat in the bath for two hours, and I pushed there for twenty-five minutes, followed by half an hour of relaxation, so three hours in all. You could refresh the water with a hose.

FRANS: The water was rather red after the delivery.

Was the placenta delivered in the water also?

PAMELA: Yes, it came about half an hour after the baby and then I got out. During the delivery, I wasn't wearing my glasses, so I didn't notice the red water. Later, when I wore them again, I didn't

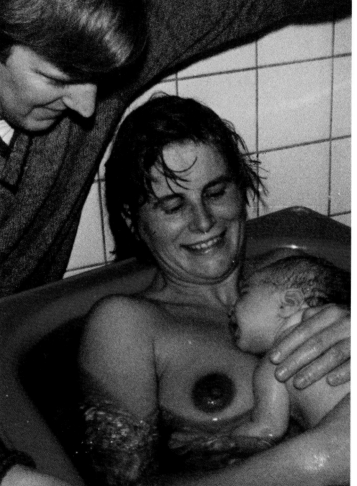

pay any attention to the color of the water; it didn't seem important enough to imprint that on my memory.

Were you scared?

FRANS: The redness was unexpected. If she had delivered traditionally, there would also have been blood. But I had seen photographs of babies delivered in tubs, in which the water remained perfectly clear.

Where were you when Pamela was in the bath?

FRANS: I sat behind the tub. She practically delivered on her own. She was seated on a bucket in the bath and started to push until the head presented itself. Beatrijs removed the bucket, and Pamela squatted, holding the edge of the bath. It didn't take long before Beatrijs brought Roland above water. He produced a sound immediately.

PAMELA: He was happy and quiet.

FRANS: Except when the midwife cleaned out his mouth and nose, which made him cry a bit. Otherwise, he was very calm.

Was he awake?

PAMELA: His eyes were closed at first. Being a mother, you think, 'I hope there are eyes behind those eyelids.'

FRANS: In the beginning, he opened and then closed them. Later on, he was fully awake. Beatrijs played with him in the bath, rocking him while he was lying on his back. He liked it a lot.

PAMELA: My most beautiful recollection of the delivery is that during the pushing, Beatrijs felt to see how far the head had descended and she allowed me to feel it, too. I felt the head, slightly rubbery and wrinkled, which was beautiful.

A little later, when Beatrijs was on the telephone, I felt the head again and noticed that it had advanced a little more. That was an amazing experience.

Did you feel close to your child during your pregnancy? Had you conjured up a picture of what Roland would look like?

I had certain feelings, but I find it hard to have contact with someone I can't see. For a long time, I had an emotional connection with him, which reached its peak in the seventh month, after which it disappeared.

When Roland was born, I couldn't do anything because I had lots of stitches to repair the perineal tears. Frans and the maternity nurse looked after the baby. His eyes moved up and down all the time as if he was searching for something. On the fifth day, when I was changing his diapers, I noticed that his eyes were less restless. And after seven days, I regained the same contact I had shared with him while he was still inside me. I thought, 'Aha, we've found each other again.'

In the first few days when I wasn't caring for him, that feeling was gone, so I am determined to do everything myself next time.

What was it like when you lost that feeling?

I was happy I had a child and everything was fine. I breastfed him, so there was some kind of contact, but not as before. I only realized this later.

Did your unborn child respond when you placed your hand on your belly?

Yes. If I had had a busy day, hardly feeling him at all, I would lie in my bed at night, thinking, 'Are you still all right?' I

would put my hand on my stomach, and he would kick as if saying, 'I am fine.' Some days I was almost unaware I was pregnant. Life just continued. I am not the type of person who needs to feel the baby three times a day.

FROM PAMELA'S DIARY: When you talk to someone, you get to know their essence. With your child, you have direct communication, as if nothing stands between you. When Roland was one week old these feelings returned. He seems a likeable person. He radiated lots of warmth toward me during the seventh month.

In me, these feelings were suppressed by my sewing urge. I had the common maternal urge to prepare everything.

Now that I am pregnant, I sense that I can develop many qualities in myself that have been dormant until now. They have more of a chance to emerge because I am closer to nature.

By the way, pregnancy has had a soothing effect on my nerves.

Does Roland still have the calming effect for you that you wrote about?

PAMELA: I am very pleased that he is here. I think he will be a support in my life and make me stronger. You carry a child, perhaps you also carry the essence of the child within you.

Before I knew I was pregnant—I hadn't done a test yet but sensed I might be pregnant—I went to the library and looked at a book with pictures of a delivery. I closed the book because I was overwhelmed. I thought that I must be pregnant for I had never reacted quite like that.

Tell me about your first contact with Roland after he was born.

FRANS: I had great difficulty understanding that he really was my child.

PAMELA: I was living in a dream. I could hardly believe my child was here. It took awhile before I accepted his presence emotionally. I was so overwhelmed that I really can't remember much of it anymore. I was filled with happiness and there wasn't

much room for other feelings. I was glad he was here and that everything had gone smoothly.

FRANS: I suspect most mothers are in a dreamworld so many things simply do not sink in.

PAMELA: I soon forgot the long labor that was just behind me, perhaps partly because I was in a daze.

FRANS: It is a pity we can't be in such a state more often. You go through a phase like that when you are madly in love. I didn't feel this at the delivery, but Pamela did. I believe too many people have boring lives, going to work in the morning and sitting in front of the television at night for years on end. Such a life does not involve many emotions. I am a mechanic and crazy about racing cars. Often, we drive to the racetrack late at night and get little sleep. When we win a twenty-four-hour race, we are exhausted but elated. Prior to such a race, I am hyped up; once you've experienced this kick, you long for it to come back. It's a kind of addiction.

Does the delivery and the contact with your child lift you out of everyday existence?

FRANS: In the beginning, I was very excited. I called several friends to describe how fabulous it was. Now, I have gone back to work and am tired at night. The baby sleeps a lot, so my interaction with her is limited, which is a pity.

What about right after the delivery?

PAMELA: When the child was born, Beatrijs told me to sit along the length of the tub, and she put him on my belly. I held him naturally, that wasn't a problem at all.

Did you feed him for the first time while you were still in the bath?

PAMELA: I breastfed him in the bath while he was still connected to me by the umbilical cord. Beatrijs instructed me to squeeze my breast somewhat so his nose would be kept free. He sucked well immediately. He has always sucked well, and the breastfeeding is going great.

Because I breastfeed him, I think he

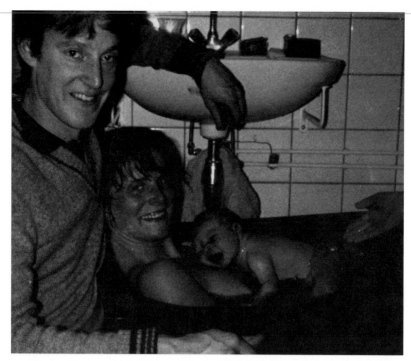

consumes what I am feeling—when I am nervous, he gets nervous, too. In this case, I give him something he doesn't need. Ideally, I would like to do everything beautifully. I am not sure that you have a similar transference when you bottle-feed a baby.

Some people claim that babies start laughing only after they are six weeks old, but Roland smiled from the beginning— the moment he enjoyed his first drops of milk and, later, during and after his meals. He still does that today. Before he smiled at me or anyone else, he had already beamed at my nipple and his milk.

Where did he spend his first night?

FRANS: We put him in a cradle that stood at the head of the bed, but we took him out and let him sleep with us most of the first two nights. In the beginning, we moved him to our bed quite often. He seemed so forlorn in that cradle, so we let him sleep in between us, feeling our warmth.

How did you feel during the first week after the delivery?

FRANS: As long as we had the assistance of the maternity nurse, visitors weren't a problem. But after she left, we found it exhausting to have guests. At times, I told Pamela, 'Please go feed him in another room because I want some sleep!' After about a month I had black circles under my eyes.

PAMELA: I enjoyed this time, especially because the maternity nurse was very friendly. This period was important to me because it is a continuation of the delivery. Physically, I was tired, but I slept in the afternoons.

Have you gone back to work?

PAMELA: When he was three months old, I went back one morning a week. I do freelance work and could decide when I wanted to start work again. To me, six weeks was far too early because I was still completely involved with my child. Things are different now. A four and a half-month-old baby is more settled in this world. It would do humankind a lot of good if the typical six-week maternity leave could be extended.

PART III

Dealing with Complications

A WOMAN MAY WISH to deliver at home but due to high blood pressure, being pregnant with twins, or the baby being in a breech position may have no choice but to deliver in a hospital. In such cases she's usually aware of her situation in advance. But because giving birth is a natural event, the course a delivery will take cannot always be predicted, and a woman who is expected to have a routine delivery may face complications. She may be admitted to the hospital shortly prior to or during the delivery because her cervix is not dilatating properly or because there are indications that the delivery may require medical intervention. A child might need to be transported to the hospital after the delivery and be put in an incubator because he or she has difficulty breathing.

The women in this section of the book encountered unexpected difficulties, and each dealt with them in her own way. Despite the setbacks, whether minor or major, they all agree that delivery as a whole, and especially the first contact with the child, was a very special, positive, and intense event. Their experiences have made them stronger and richer people.

JOSÉ AND PAUL

José: Linda's mother
Linda: firstborn, a girl (born at home, taken to hospital)
Paul: Linda's father
Nicolientje: neighbor's daughter
Marijke: neighbor
Nora: a girlfriend
Astrid: midwife

THIS INTERVIEW TOOK PLACE ELEVEN WEEKS AFTER LINDA'S BIRTH.

Did your career as a general practitioner, and especially your experience with deliveries, influence your decision to have a home delivery?

JOSÉ: Experiences in my work have caused me to develop an aversion to hospitals, so I was highly motivated to deliver at home. In my opinion, too much unnecessary intervention takes place in a hospital. Part of my training during internship was to assist at medically intervened deliveries, and I was surprised at the high percentage of births that this included. Only later did I realize that in many cases that intervention had not been required and hadn't been pleasant for the women involved. I have never encountered anything really upsetting, like congenital abnormalities or an enormously difficult labor. Last year all the home deliveries I attended went very smoothly. I always went enthusiastically to these deliveries because they were cozy and I enjoyed conducting them.

Giving birth yourself must be quite different?

I had completely visualized how I wanted to do delivery—sitting vertically on a bucket. I had chosen which part of the house, and had pictured Paul sitting behind me, but I could not imagine the pain that accompanied the contractions. I had never experienced severe pain in my life. At the deliveries I conducted, I always found it hard to empathize with what the woman was feeling during contractions. I wonder to what extent this influenced my actions as I stood next to the woman's bed.

How did you come to decide to deliver vertically?

I have only assisted at horizontal deliveries. Agaath, a midwife, told me about this option, and although vertical birth interested me, at first I found it an odd concept, which is a natural reaction when all you've ever known about is horizontal delivery. I thought about it for a couple of weeks, and then I had to admit it was more logical to make use of gravity. If she had waited to suggest it until during the delivery, I wouldn't have complied and would have remained supine because fear of the unknown would have prevailed.

Your girlfriend, your sister, and the neighbor and her young daughter were present at your delivery. What was it like to be surrounded by this many people?

It was extremely comforting. They sat opposite me so I could see them all very well. Nora would wink at me, which was quite encouraging. Astrid supported and praised me again and again, making comments like 'Things are advancing well. You are doing fine.'

What was it like to have a four-year-old girl present?

I was taken aback when Marijke asked me if Nicolientje could remain there. I didn't know whether this was a good idea. Later, I got used to it. I thought as long as Marijke approved that was her business. Somebody asked the midwife, 'Do you think a child that young can cope with it?' Astrid replied, 'You can count on children to walk away if something is too much for them to handle.' So she stayed. I enjoyed Nicolientje's presence. She often stole the show because her reactions were so pure. She crawled onto everybody's laps, and made the most poignant comments. Just as Linda was about to be born, Nicolientje whispered to Astrid, 'we are going to help.' She sat arm in arm with Astrid in front of me, and the two of them were so charming. When Linda was born, Nicolientje was remarkably helpful and highly interested in the baby. We've got a few slides in which she's cleaning up some blood with a cloth.

Has Nicolientje talked about the birth?

Last Thursday, she came by with some of her girlfriends and presented Linda with one of her own dolls. I heard from Marijke that Nicolientje told her classmates that she had seen a delivery where there was lots of blood, but that was all that was said.

Did you enjoy sitting on the bucket?

Very much. Before I sat on the bucket, I sat on the sofa and pushed, which felt strange because I couldn't put what I was pushing against into perspective. I leaned backwards, but on the bucket I bent forward.

Did you feel you could cope with the birth process?

I felt very involved until the child was born. I was exhausted. A few hours earlier I had already hoped everything would go faster because I was getting tired. Concentrating on my contractions took a lot out of me, and after that I had to push the baby out.

Was it difficult to remain active when you were already tired?

Yes. Even when I was ready to push, I would have preferred to sigh the urge away. Then I thought I might be able to push beyond the pain. Although I pushed diligently three or four times—taking in some extra air and sustaining the effort—I still couldn't overcome the pain.

How did you feel immediately after Linda was born?

Relief that I had managed to squeeze her out of my big belly was the most predominant feeling. I was too drained to push anymore. It never really seemed as if I had been pushing out a child, a human being. Later, I felt rather bad about my initial reaction—it seemed so selfish. But I realize that exhaustion played a major part in how I felt.

PAUL: Another factor may be that Linda didn't cry much. Had she done so, she might have evoked a stronger reaction from you.

JOSÉ: I think you are right. What was I to respond to in the first moments after the birth when she was just a groaning creature? Astrid said, 'Why don't you say something to the baby? She will react to you.' Mechanically, as if a switch had been turned on, I uttered, 'Linda, Linda.' I did that only because I was told to, not because it come from my heart. Things would have been different if Linda had appealed to me by crying or had looked at me intently. I had imagined that I would be very emotional when she arrived, but this didn't happen until the following day. Linda was still in the incubator, but she was doing well. She was hungry, and I put her to my breast. That is the moment you really become aware that you have a child.

PAUL: I was surprised that Linda reacted when José called out her name. She opened her eyes, and I thought, 'Gosh, it works.'

How much time did Linda spend in the hospital?

JOSÉ: Almost four days—from Saturday morning to Wednesday afternoon. Because of my profession, I should have seen that Linda wasn't breathing properly, but it never really sank in. Astrid saw the problem immediately and recommended that we see a pediatrician if her condition did not improve. I looked more closely and, indeed, judging from Linda's nostrils, saw that she had breathing difficulties. I was still far too hazy for it to dawn on me that she might be admitted to a hospital.

Did Linda's health improve quickly?

On Sunday I visited her twice. Linda

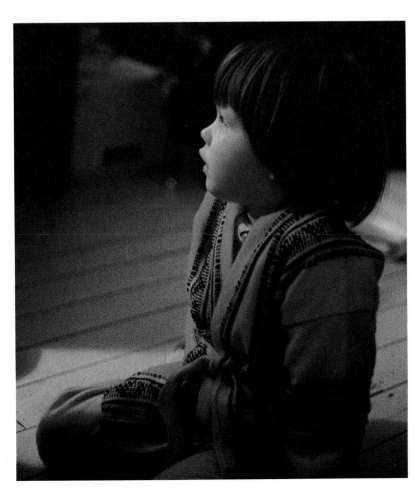

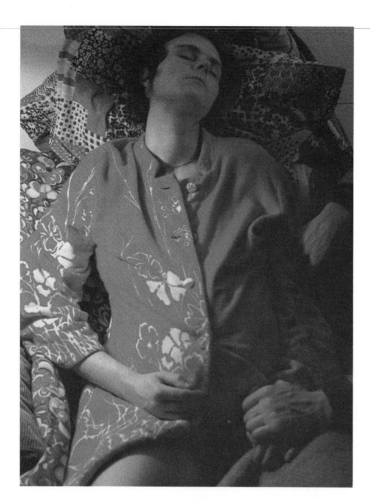

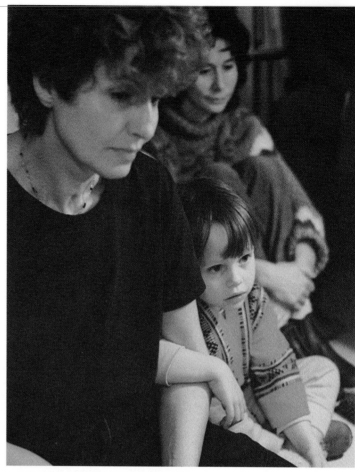

looked rosy and was screaming like a real baby. I asked immediately if I could breastfeed her. Feeding went well, and I became very emotional and felt my warmth go out to her. She was still in the incubator with extra oxygen. Originally, they had put a cap on her head, which supplied her with exactly the amount of oxygen she needed. By Sunday night, she was in a cradle. The only reason she continued to stay in the hospital was because she was taking antibiotics. We were told at first that she'd have to stay for two weeks. I couldn't believe my ears and wondered how I could ever continue to breastfeed her. We traveled back and forth between the hospital and home all that time, which was terribly exhausting.

PAUL: When Linda was given to me right after the delivery my first thought was that she was a real child. Saliva was coming from her mouth, but I thought little of it. When it was decided that she should go into the hospital, I felt it was probably a good idea. In the hospital, I watched them put tubes into her and give her injections. I waited until the x-rays had been taken before I returned home and slept for a while. Back home, I was overwhelmed by tears. I comforted myself by saying that this was part of it and would soon pass, but when I saw all those people in white coats working with sterile equipment, it suddenly dawned on me, 'My goodness, who knows what is in store for us,' and I felt utterly lost.

It must have been strange for the two of you to come home without the baby.

JOSÉ: Yes, you wonder what you sat up for all night. You feel wronged because you have worked hard and still don't have your child. The first things that went through my mind were: What is wrong with her? How long is this going to last? Will this have lifelong repercussions: I was afraid that the lack of oxygen may have caused irreversible brain damage. I was frightened about Linda's future and was restless because she was away from me in an incubator. But when I saw her again on Sunday, I realized she was going to be all right, although she still had a drip in her arm and had to finish the round of antibiotics she was on. It was very important for me to be with her, especially in those first few days. My stitches stung and pulled so much at one point that I didn't know how to sit on those terrible hospital chairs. I always ached whether I sat on the right or left buttock. On Monday night I was changing her diaper. As I was bending down, I realized I was dead tired, and I almost passed out! When she came home, we were flooded with visitors, so I was utterly worn out by the fifth or sixth day.

What was it like to have Linda home?

PAUL: That week I was mighty busy pouring coffee, changing diapers and doing the shopping, and José was having problems with her stitches.

JOSÉ: I didn't seem to be successful at breastfeeding Linda, and it hurt. But I was determined and carried on. And all those

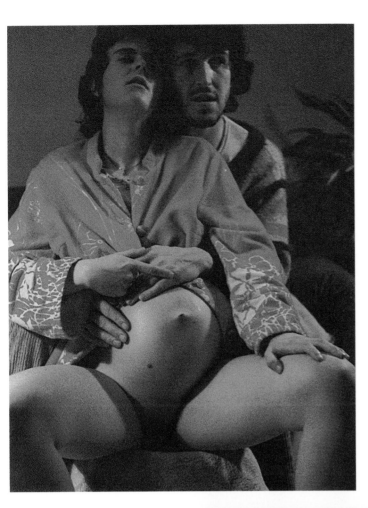
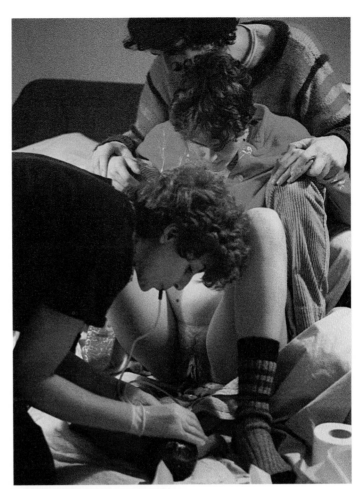
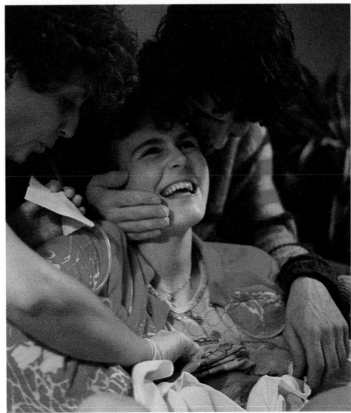

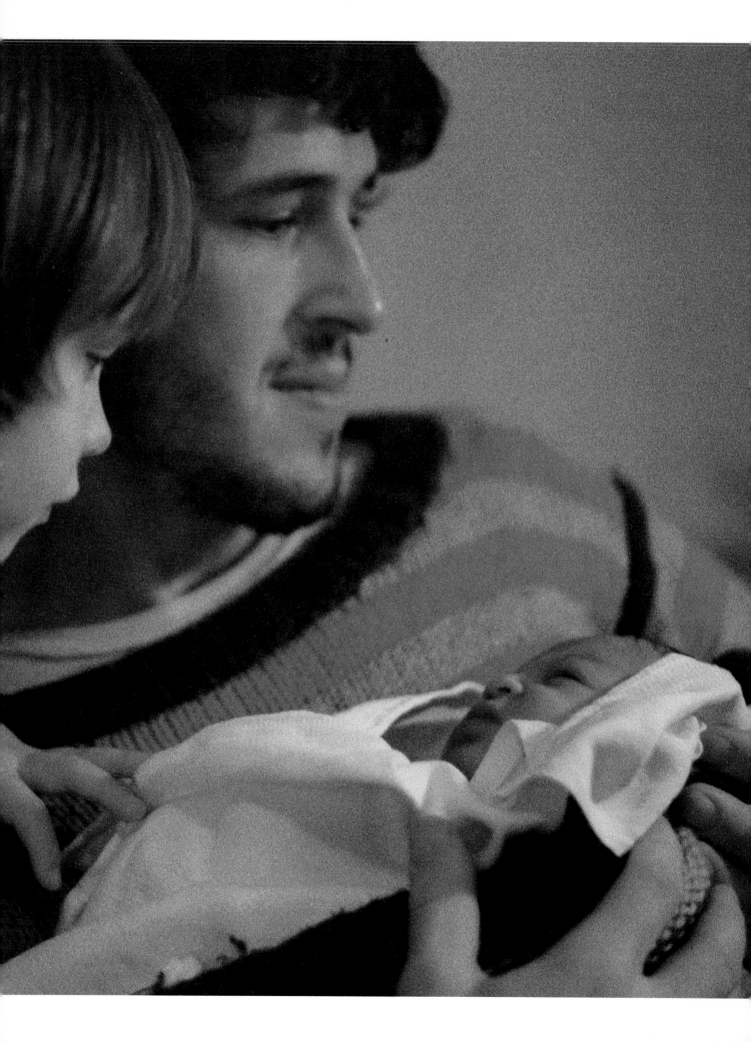

visitors! And those stitches! And still losing blood! I took countless showers to keep the stitches as clean as possible. I had no time for myself or to establish contact with Linda.

José, you've had quite limited experience with babies. Did you know how to hold her immediately?

Perhaps holding your own baby is an instinctive talent mothers have because I feel less comfortable holding someone else's baby. During the home deliveries I attended, either the midwife or I would catch the baby and hand it to the mother. I remember feeling as though I had two left hands because I'd had no experience with newborns, so the midwife preferred to do it herself because she was much quicker. I've never really held many babies. When I see my girlfriend's babies I just look. Many of my friends and acquaintances wanted to hold Linda, which was all right with me, but I never felt inclined to do so with other babies.

Do you feel Linda has changed your lives?

JOSÉ: During pregnancy I felt very calm. Other people commented on this also.

PAUL: That shouldn't surprise you. It's not as if magic is involved in calming down pregnant women. It has more to do with having a clearly defined goal at the end of a predictable amount of time.

JOSÉ: You also go through a lot of hormonal changes during pregnancy, and now that I am breastfeeding, I am influenced by different hormones. But unfortunately, I have lost my calm. It is hard to define my feelings for Linda. I am proud of her. I have compared her to other babies, and, naturally, she comes off most favorably. Just the same, I have to get used to the idea that she is my daughter; I still don't quite know what that implies. Motherhood does not seem to suit me yet; I am still more the old José than the person I sense I shall become. Part of the reason I don't know what my maternal feelings are is because I am still working. I

feel I need more practice; but as time goes on, Linda means more and more to me. Sometimes I get these flashes that she is no longer with us, and I panic completely.

PAUL: I want Linda to change my life and am looking forward to contributing a great deal to her upbringing.

JOSÉ: We share an affection toward Linda, who is now the focus of our attention. We have a lot of fun with the baby. Through her eyes, we will rediscover the world and relive our own childhoods. Having a child as the link changes a relationship. We hardly kiss each other these days. It would have been hard for me to imagine this would happen. Naturally, things between Paul and I will change, but that is unavoidable. Some things are lost, which is sad, but Linda has become an integral part of our lives and will always be there. When the three of us sit together, a warmth radiates among us.

META

Meta: Jeffrey's mother
Jeffrey: first child, a boy (born in hospital)
Bob: Jeffrey's father
Agaath: midwife

THIS INTERVIEW TOOK PLACE THREE MONTHS AFTER JEFFREY'S BIRTH.

How did you react to the news that you had to go to the hospital because your efforts to deliver at home were not successful?

META: I asked to be taken to hospital. I even asked for a Cesarean section, which they didn't do, because I realized that no progress had been made. I had tried everything: pushing on the bucket in the sitting position, on my knees, and standing.

When I was standing, Bob supported me with his arms, but he didn't seem to have enough strength to hold me, which made me feel insecure. Bob is a fairly strong man, so you can imagine the kind of power you have in you at such a time. Kneeling on the floor while bending forward onto the bed was not a bad position, but because Jeffrey didn't descend fast enough, I knew that pushing in this position would not be effective either. I had no strength left, and I was troubled by terrible back-

aches. In an attempt to relieve the pain, they put hot-water bottles on my back and massaged me.

What happened after you decided to go to the hospital?

The ambulance arrived, and I walked downstairs by myself. I laid down on the stretcher and was driven to hospital where I was taken quickly to the delivery room. I believe the doctor was about to introduce himself to me when I interrupted

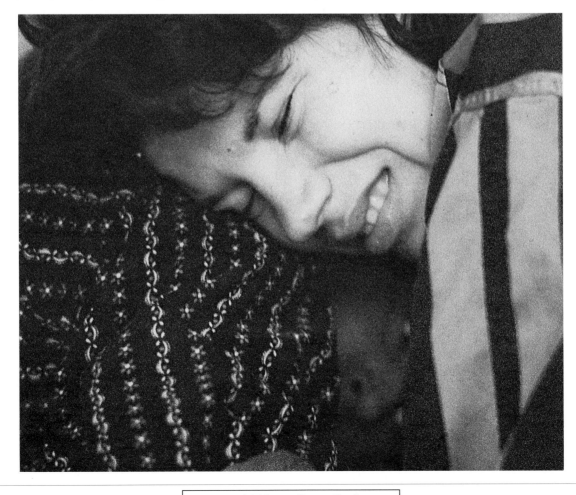

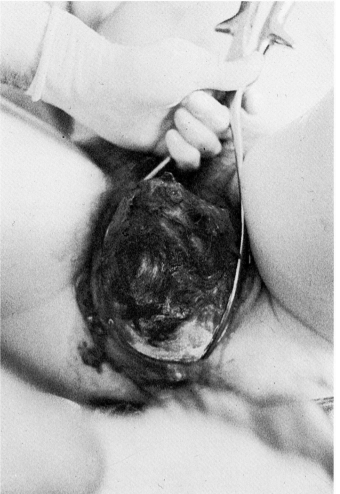

him and said something like, 'Please do everything as quickly as possible.' At one point, I asked what they were going to do, and they told me it would be a forceps delivery. All I wanted was to be delivered because I was getting fed up with the situation.

They asked me whether I wanted an anesthetic. I suffered intolerable pain despite the anesthetic. The contractions were agonizing, and I was very sore when they inserted the forceps. I felt like the whole area was being stretched. Afterwards, I noticed that when I stood or sat in a certain position, I'd feel incredible pressure on my pubic bone, which most likely was caused by the forceps. I never felt the episiotomy because the anesthetic had numbed my vagina. The stitching did not hurt either; well, perhaps the last stitch hurt a little bit because the anesthetic had worn off.

The people in the hospital were very kind and spent time with me to help me cope with the situation. I was happy to stay in hospital after the delivery. Jeffrey did not sleep in my room the first night. I was dead tired and relieved that I did not have to take care of my child in my own house that first night because I was still confused. Visitors would have been flooding into the house continually; here, there were visiting hours and I had a whole array of people around my bed for two hours, but then it would be quiet again.

During labor, were you aware of your surroundings?

I was totally absorbed in myself. It wouldn't have bothered me if ten people had been there. You don't hear them because you are the one who has to do the job. No one can do the work for you, and in that sense, you are quite alone. Others may whisper encouraging words, but they can't take away the pain.

In the final stages of the dilatation, I was in agony, but now I can't recall that pain. I can certainly remember the moment that Jeffrey was put on my belly. I was washed and taken back into the ward, and someone carried him in front of me. Back on the ward, I ate the traditional birth biscuits and felt incredibly proud. 'I have accomplished it,' I thought. Although I hadn't slept all night, I wasn't the least bit tired.

What was Bob's experience of the birth?

Although I have asked him from time to time, he is rather reluctant to talk about it. Bob cried when Jeffrey was born, and I was in tears watching him cry. He is as proud as a peacock and really enjoys having a child. If Jeffrey goes for a day without smiling at him, Bob is quite upset about it.

Did the stitches bother you later?

Not really. I had a stinging sensation from time to time, but it wasn't painful. However, after three months, I am still a bit incontinent and need to wear a pad. At the end of the day, when I am tired, I lose control, which is a nuisance. I see a physiotherapist, who is instructing me how to exercise the muscles of the pelvic floor. Even before my pregnancy, I found it hard to hold my urine when laughing or sneezing, so my muscles have never been really strong. But he agrees that the forceps might be the main reason it is so lax now that I can't control it. I am working hard to tighten the muscle again. Sometimes I get a nasty, itchy feeling that might have been caused by the forceps as well.

What went through your mind the first moment you saw Jeffrey?

It took a moment before I realized it was my child. My initial reaction was surprise about his weight. He screeched at the top of his lungs. He opened his eyes immediately, which was marvelous. I found my baby so beautiful, with dark hair and those fierce, big eyes.

Did you talk to him?

Yes, I welcomed him. Jeffrey looked at me as if he could see, and there was an immediate bond between us. Last Sunday, I watched a delivery on TV, and when the baby was given to its mother, she merely watched it. I thought, 'Come on, talk to it.'

What was life like when you returned home?

I returned home on a Tuesday and had my first crying fit that night. I didn't find this out until later, but my mother-in-law told everybody who called her not to visit me the first week because I had had such a difficult time. In the first week just family members visited us; in the second, third, and fourth weeks, I was extremely busy entertaining friends.

Though my life has changed from one day to the next, in the last two weeks I have been feeling a bit more myself and have begun to see things more the way I used to. I often feel insecure and think that breastfeeding has something to do with it.

Will you go back to work?

No, I want to spend lots of time with Jeffrey. I am going to play with him and do exercises to stimulate his development. In the first few weeks, I felt rather disillusioned—all I did was feed him, after which I put him back in his crib. I did not like that at all. It is much more fun now.

When did you start enjoying Jeffrey more?

When he began to smile. I had some kind of contact with him when he was small, but it was less defined. Now I can really play with him, and the contact between us is just incredible. If I were to put him in his crib right now and do nothing, he would make sounds and would look at me as if saying, 'I want to play again,' and I would continue my games with him.

Does Bob play with Jeffrey?

The older Jeffrey is, the more Bob enjoys playing with him. Jeffrey did not really respond to Bob in the beginning. When Jeffrey responds to him, Bob is ecstatic and their contact is very natural. Last week, Bob was taking a bath. Jeffrey was dirty and needed a bath. I told Bob, 'Don't make the water too hot because Jeffrey is joining you.' He muttered a few objections, but I told him not to make a fuss. Well, I handed Jeffrey to him and said, 'Relax, Bob. If you hold on to him, nothing can happen.' The both loved it. I sprinkled water over Jeffrey while Bob was holding him. It was lovely. I took some photos. I want it to happen more often.

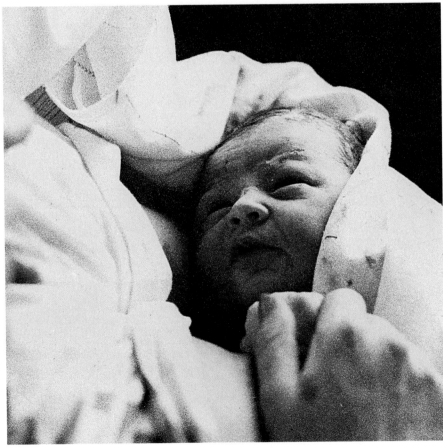

RIET

Riet: Harm's mother
Harm: second child, a boy (born in hospital)
Hetty: firstborn, a girl (born in hospital)
Harry: Harm's father

THIS INTERVIEW TOOK PLACE EIGHT MONTHS AFTER HARM'S BIRTH.

Tell me about the complications of your first pregnancy.

RIET: In the beginning, I had idealistic visions of a home delivery. I was seeing a midwife, but when I was five months pregnant, things started to go wrong—my blood pressure rose. I was admitted to hospital when I was seven months along and remained there for two months. I was told to stay in bed, and all those beautiful dreams of delivery seemed very far away. I was tense and worried about what lay ahead. It was also difficult for Harry who was at home alone. At the hospital, we had no privacy—we were constantly surrounded by other people.

I had been admitted to the hospital because of high blood pressure. I didn't anticipate that it would come to a Cesarean section. But the child wouldn't grow due to the elevated blood pressure, and in such a case, a Cesarean is indicated. After they told me I'd have to have a Cesarean, I sometimes thought, 'Just go on and get her.' On January 9, the doctor came to my bed and told me that I would be delivered the next day.

Were you overdue?

No, Hetty was due on the 18th, but her condition had deteriorated. They could tell from my urine that the baby wasn't taking enough food, so they decided she should be born immediately.

Were you depressed during your hospital stay?

I had days, moments rather, when I felt I was up against a wall. Usually, I'd take a shower, cry my eyes out, and feel better afterwards. One of the many uses of water.

What happened when Hetty was delivered?

I had prepared myself for her to be tiny. At a certain point, I surrendered completely to the gynecologist's expertise because I couldn't do anything myself anyway. But I did ask whether Harry could stay with me during the surgery, which wasn't allowed. He was given permission to keep me company while I was given a sedative to make me sleep before I was wheeled into the delivery room.

When we approached the swinging doors of the operating room, which had a sign that said 'forbidden to the public,' she pushed me and my bed through.

Harry, not knowing what to do, came along. At the very last moment, the nurse turned around and said, 'Sorry, sorry, but you can't come along.' Harry kissed me and wished me well, and the nurse closed the door on him. It was a horrendous experience. I waited for what seemed ages, though actually, it wasn't very long. I was shivering from increasing fear and because the operating room was awfully cold. Then they moved me under big, bright lights and put the necessary drips into my arm. The doctor arrived, wished me well, and I was gone into oblivion.

Did you have any choice about being put under general anesthesia?

From the moment they told me the delivery would be Cesarean, I was frightened out of my wits. I was unaware of alternatives to being put under and simply acquiesced to the doctor's decision without questioning anything.

Did they tell you how long you would be anesthetized?

They could not give me a definite answer because everybody responds differently. I remember coming around, and the nurse said that I had a daughter. I asked her whether Harry had already been informed of the good news. While I had been out of it two hours had passed, so naturally he already knew. In fact, many people knew because Harry had called my mother and mother-in-law immediately when he heard the child was healthy.

When did you get to see Hetty?

The moment I came around. Although I dozed off occasionally due to the aftereffects of the anesthetic, I was convinced I was wide awake. In any event, they wheeled my bed to the incubator ward.

What was it like when you saw her?

Tears ran down my cheeks. I heard the nurse exclaim, 'She is so happy,' but her voice seemed to come from very far away. Hetty's face seemed blurred, with the exception of her eyes, which were wide open. I saw her big, clear eyes but couldn't really make out her face.

How much distance was between you and your child?

About ten feet. My bed was a yard or so in front of the window dividing us, and on the other side, nurses held her up about two yards away from the window. I was overjoyed nevertheless. I can't tell you how happy I was. Especially because they had warned me before the Cesarean that my expectation should not be too high as things might go wrong. I had prepared myself for a total letdown, and then I heard my child was alive and saw her in front of me.

Was Hetty all right?

She breathed immediately so I was reassured that her lungs functioned, but she was awfully skinny. The doctor told us we shouldn't send any birth announcements yet, which upset me terribly. After a day had passed, I asked the head nurse of the pediatric ward if Hetty was making any progress and explained to her our anxiety about the announcements. She answered laconically, 'Oh, they can be sent. She has started to grow already.'

We were overjoyed of course. The following Monday, the gynecologist visited me and saw the birth announcements. Believing he showed a personal interest when he asked about them, I handed him one immediately. 'But,' he continued, 'hasn't the pediatrician told you that you should wait with that?' I would have preferred to have been hit on the head by a hammer than to hear that. It shows how little communication there was between the people caring for us. When Harry came by during visiting hours, I was in tears. He questioned all the staff involved and apparently everything was fine.

When were you allowed to have Hetty with you?

In the beginning when I stood in front of that window, I accepted everything. I wanted to touch her but didn't feel strong enough to ask for permission. As long as I was timid and compliant, the nurses were helpful and informed me enthusiastically about Hetty's progress. However, the moment I showed any initiative and insisted that I wanted to hold my baby, they ignored me completely. I believe they considered me a troublesome mother. When I objected, I was told that I was unstable and emotional from the

delivery. Well, I was 'unstable and emotional' for thirteen solid days until I finally had her in my arms.

Why did they make you wait so long?

We made quite a fuss. Harry regularly visited the pediatrician who told him that as soon as Hetty weighed 4 pounds, 6 ounces, she'd be allowed out of isolation. She'd be put into a specially heated room where we could touch her. Every day we asked how much weight she had gained. One afternoon, the scale read 4 pounds, 7½ ounces. We looked forward excitedly to when she would be released from her incubator. But she wasn't moved at all that afternoon. I told Harry to go to the pediatrician because by then, the nurses were snubbing me all the time, and I wasn't willing to ask them anything. The doctor agreed that Hetty could be moved and called the pediatric ward. Harry heard the nurses object to the pediatrician's instructions until he said, 'Yes, you heard me; she is allowed out.'

Harry returned in a good mood and described to me what had happened. When visiting hour was over, I went upstairs with leaden feet. She had been taken out of her incubator. I expected someone to be there who would say, 'Come, you may touch her and hold her now,' but there was absolutely no one in sight. I wept and felt inconsolably sad. I went downstairs in search of one of the staff nurses. I poured out my heart to her once more, and she promised to discuss the matter with the other staff nurse. After that, we finally made an appointment to take our daughter in our arms.

What was it like to finally hold her?

I enjoyed it, of course, but she was totally wrapped up in many layers of cloth. No skin-to-skin contact was possible. Her face was the only part of her visible. I had never seen her face so close. After a bit, we unwrapped her some because her arms were entirely swaddled the way they used to do it in the old days.

How many times a day were you allowed to hold her?

I could look at her from behind the window as often as I wanted, but I could only hold her once a day. Their timetable was obviously more important than my feelings. In my opinion, they know nothing about feelings. But getting angry didn't help; in fact, it only made things worse. At one point, the nurses refused to come near me. Harry, who has a calmer disposition, said, 'Let it go, we are going to have her home soon.' I resigned myself to the situation, but deep down, I was furious.

You took her home when she was about six weeks old?

They promised us she could leave the hospital when she weighed five pounds. So Harry and I impatiently awaited the day she reached that weight, which, compared to other premature babies, was rather early.

What was it like to finally have her home?

Great, but it took a lot of getting used to because she screamed form early in the morning until late at night. Her crying worried me, and she sensed this, which made her worse. It was a vicious circle. This tense situation lasted seven weeks; I'll never forget it because I almost went mad. Sometimes I was at my wits' end. I had fed her and her diapers were clean. In desperation, I would change her pants again. It was midwinter and ice cold. I was not allowed to take her outside until she had had her six-week checkup after her release from hospital. I felt suffocated.

Sometimes, in desperation, I called someone for help to ask what I should do with her. I tried everything. I put her in the living room…in the kitchen…but she never calmed down unless I held her close to me. She was fine the moment I took her into my arms. Visitors would say that I spoiled her and should just let her cry. That advice made me feel insecure because I had conflicting emotions. They were trying to be helpful, but I am glad I let her be close to me and did not let her cry. In retrospect, I realize we all had to get used to each other, but at the time I was unaware of that.

By seven o'clock at night, she had exhausted herself so she slept soundly through the night. We enjoyed a good night's rest, but at 6:30 A.M., she would start crying again. Unless I held her in my arms, she'd weep all day long. Naturally, I couldn't hold her the whole day because I had housework and errands to do. When I left her with someone while I went shopping, her cry would continue to ring in my head and almost drove me insane. Harry came home at five o'clock. When we had finished our dinner, I fed her and put her to bed because she was totally exhausted. Harry didn't quite know what it meant to be with a crying child all day. Except for weekends, he wasn't around when she was awake, and when both of us looked after her—which Hetty enjoyed thoroughly—things were different.

How did your second pregnancy go?

I had a miscarriage at four and a half months. I went in for my regular checkup, and the midwife wanted to listen to the heart tones. She heard nothing, though I was sixteen weeks pregnant. An ultrasound made it clear that the fetus was not alive and had to be removed. My belly was still growing, and I felt very pregnant, and proud of it, not knowing there wasn't really a child in me. Apparently, it probably lived for only five weeks, but the doctors couldn't judge this very accurately because it had already decayed considerably. I was aborted in June, and the following January I conceived again.

Was that pregnancy normal?

I didn't dare count on anything anymore. I was happy when the first three months passed without any complications and was relieved to hear the heartbeat clearly, though I was painfully reminded of my miscarriage. When I was four months pregnant, I decided to stick to a salt-free diet and got into the habit of taking a nap in the afternoon when I put Hetty down. The pregnancy didn't seem like nine months because I slept more than I was awake. The child was growing, and I had no complications.

On my due date, I was lying in bed when the contractions began. I said, 'Harry, this is the beginning.' I was thrilled. Every half hour, I would have a special sensation. At a certain point, I felt it come more frequently. I told Harry to go back to sleep; I would wake him if necessary. I just laid there watching the clock. When five minutes had passed and nothing happened, I was enraged at the situation and at Harry for not waking up, even though I had instructed him to go to sleep. I called the hospital because I was worried, and the chief nurse of the obstetric ward told me to stay put.

Another week elapsed, and during my last regular checkup, the baby's heartbeat was not good. I told Harry that I preferred to go to a different hospital because I was afraid of another incubator disaster, but on the other hand, I had liked the gynecologist—he really took the time to listen to my experiences when Hetty was born. We chose to return to the hospital we had used when Hetty was born, but I decided that were I to have another Cesarean section, I'd prefer local anesthesia to general.

Where had you heard about that option?

A friend of mind had her first baby under a local. The anesthetist came to see me the evening before the Cesarean to get my medical history. He was very supportive of my decision to have an epidural. He told me that if his wife ever needed a Cesarean section, they would opt for an epidural. Hospital regulations had changed since Hetty was born, and Harry was allowed to be present while the anesthetic was put into my spine. I didn't feel its effects for one and a half hours. Harry wasn't allowed to attend the actual operation, but he didn't want to see me cut open anyway.

To what extent were you aware of what was happening to you during the operation?

I didn't feel any pain, I didn't feel the incision, yet I was not entirely without sensation—I felt them fiddling away. It is like being anesthetized by a dentist, where you are not completely numbed either. A rack with a sheet over it was put up so I couldn't see my tummy, which I didn't mind at all.

At a certain point, I overheard the anesthetist say, 'goddamn it, this incision is too small,' and I shivered from excitement rather than from fear. They had difficulty getting the baby out because they had just reopened the incision that had been made to deliver my tiny Hetty, which proved to be too small now, so they had to make it larger. The gynecologist asked to assist the anesthetist because he couldn't get the child out by himself. He had to push on my belly, which didn't hurt but did create some pressure. I really liked the anesthetist because he looked very much like Harry—he had the same kind of beard—so I pretended that it was Harry who helped the baby be born.

I felt the baby being taken out of me, and then they gave me my son, which was lovely. After a moment, the nurse took him away, which infuriated the anesthetist. But I was happy. All I was interested in was knowing how much Harm weighed. I still dreaded the possibility of the incubator and was thrilled when I heard he weighed six and a half pounds.

What happened then?

I wanted the nurse to give Harm back to me, but that wasn't allowed. The anesthetist claimed it was quite unnecessary that the nurse took the baby away so quickly. The baby, accompanied by Harry, was wheeled off to the obstetrics ward in a mobile incubator. Harry was allowed to hold Harm right away. Together, the nurse and he tested Harm's reflexes.

In the meantime, I was still in the operating room because I needed to be stitched up. The anesthetist asked whether I wanted to have a general anesthetic; I didn't because I was afraid I might be unconscious for quite a long time. It took awhile, but when I was sewed up, the nurse transferred me to the obstetrics ward and the baby was given to me immediately. His cradle was placed next to my bed. So many things about the hospital had changed within just a couple of years. Before, even mothers with uncomplicated deliveries hadn't been allowed to have their babies next to them. When the drips had been removed from my arm, I was free to move as I liked. Despite my stitches I could walk in and out of the nursery. If Harm was in the nursery and I heard him cry, I could go in to change his diaper or feed him without asking anybody's permission. I insisted on breastfeeding him. The moment I put him to my breast, he drank beautifully. The drips delayed milk production somewhat during the first few days, but after that, feeding went well. The nurses were amused at how I applied myself to breastfeeding heart and soul.

Why were you given a drip after the surgery?

It contained antibiotics to prevent the wound from becoming infected.

Did Harm lean against your stitches when you breastfed him?

Yes, but it didn't bother me. The incision only hurt when I burst out laughing. One day, lots of friends came to visit me, and we were all laughing. Tears partly from pleasure and partly because of the pain, ran down my face.

What was it like to bring Harm home?

We stayed in hospital for two weeks. Everything went beautifully when we got home because Harm hadn't been deprived of contact. He used to wake up during the night quite often, but after I fed him, he'd go back to sleep again.

Hetty loves him madly, and so far, I have noticed no signs of jealousy. When I feed Harm, she strokes his head with one hand while she sucks the thumb of her other hand. Hetty is very quiet, but Harm is a ball of energy who could already stand up at only seven months.

How did people react to the fact you had had a Cesarean section?

Close family and friends were supportive and understood my disappointment that I couldn't have the normal delivery for which I had hoped. Six to ten people whom I know only superficially made comments such as, 'Oh, that's the easy way'; 'I wouldn't mind delivering that way'; and 'So you never suffered from contractions'; and 'That's how princesses deliver.' Indirectly they accused me of having chosen the easy way out without having any idea what a Cesarean entails.

MIEKE

Mieke: Kyra's mother
Kyra: first child, a girl (born in hospital)
Gauke: Kyra's father
Beatrijs and Astrid: midwives
Henriette: midwife trainee

THIS INTERVIEW TOOK PLACE FOUR WEEKS AFTER KYRA'S BIRTH.

Before you found out that Kyra may be breech, how much did you know about breech deliveries?

MIEKE: I knew very little. I had read a bit about it, but Beatrijs told me all the details. She explained that breech babies must be born much more quickly because of the increased chance of the umbilical cord getting squashed, cutting off the child's source of oxygen. She also said that since the biggest part of the baby, the head, comes out last, it is important that the dilatation is absolutely complete. After that appointment, I went home and rummaged through magazines in search of photographs of breech deliveries.

Beatrijs couldn't be sure if the child was lying in the breech position—it was hard for her to tell because I have a very muscley belly—so she referred me to a gynecologist, who would do an ultrasound.

What did the ultrasound show?

The moment the gy-necologist put the instrument on my tummy, he exclaimed, 'This is plainly a breech.' Hearing this, I broke into a cold sweat. He pointed out the skull, spine, heart, of which I could make out nothing; then, suddenly, we saw the contours of a hand crystal clear, a fist that opened

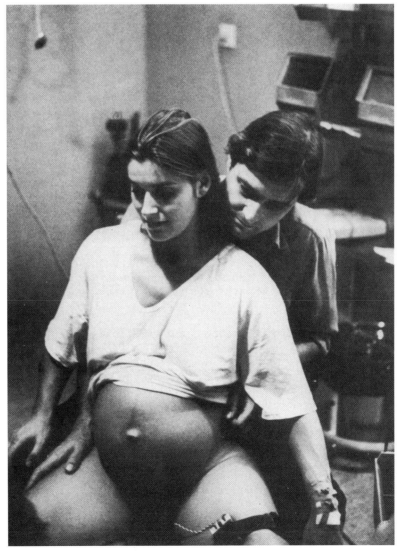

and seemed to wave before it closed again. The baby was so real and so human suddenly.

How was the experience of dealing with hospital personnel different from the interactions you had had with your midwives up until that time?

I didn't like the atmosphere of the hospital when we went for the ultrasound. Women in white coats were running around, or shouted from behind the counter, 'Have you got your white card? Have you got any urine? Here's a bottle, there's the bathroom.'

I was astounded and knew I didn't want to deliver in a place like that. We had to wait our turn, and it really bothered me how they called out my name from the distance. The nurse shook my hand only and then led the way into the room. Gauke dragged behind me like a dog. During the conference about the results, which proved she was breech, Gauke was left out. He sat in the corner. I tried to involve him in the conversation but wasn't successful because I was so nervous about the results. In my opinion,

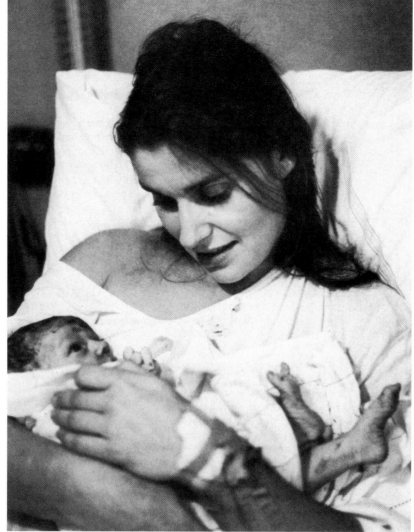

men are too often left in the dark in a hospital. With Beatrijs and Agaath, the situation was completely different. They asked him as many questions as they asked me.

Had you tried to imagine what the delivery would be like?

My image of the delivery was very vague. I had no concrete idea how Gauke and I would react to each other, how we'd cope with the contractions, but I was positive that I didn't want to deliver lying down. Beatrijs recommended some books, but sadly enough, I never read them. Perhaps I was avoiding the issue, though I discussed it with many people, who invariably had sisters or grandchildren who had delivered breech—all without any problems. I didn't hear one negative story. One woman told me that her firstborn had been a complicated normal delivery but her second child was born very smoothly in the breech position. I was encouraged by these stories and felt little inclination to read more about it.

Why were you so sure that you didn't want to be supine?

During one of the first consultations, Beatrijs asked me how I wanted to deliver. I told her I wanted to be at home so I could walk around. Beatrijs explained sev-eral possible birthing positions, including sitting and standing. I wanted to sit. It seemed logical that being upright would help the child come out.

How did your labor begin?

Cervical dilatation lasted forty-nine hours. I had severe contractions every five minutes. It all started in bed. We'd gone to bed at midnight, and I woke up half an hour later thinking I had to go to the bathroom. Within two hours, the contractions were so powerful that I knew I was in labor. I walked around the house and hung onto Gauke or the kitchen sink. It was impossible to handle the contractions sitting in a chair. My favorite position was to lean with both arms on the kitchen sink while rounding my back so the front part of me could relax and I could breathe properly.

Had you practiced breathing techniques?

I went to a pregnancy course four times, and it was useful for the breathing exercises. I concentrated on short inspirations and long expirations for quite awhile at the beginning, which helped distract me from the pain. When the labor first started, I had no idea what was going to lie ahead, but I wasn't worried. I still answered phone calls. The further into the labor, the less interested I became in my immediate surroundings.

Finally, upon Beatrijs's recommendation, I got into the tub. She said it would stimulate the contractions, and I enjoyed it tremendously. I sat in the bath most of the rest of the time I was home. By 6:00 A.M. after my second night of labor, the cervix had not dilatated more than one centimeter. At four the following afternoon, we went to the hospital. By that time, the dilatation was six to seven centimeters.

The move to the hospital changed the situation quite a bit, didn't it?

It was so strange, almost cartoonish. I realized I had to get dressed to go to the hospital. It seemed like so much work to find a sweater and a pair of pants. It was raining cats and dogs. I saw nothing on the way there because I was concentrat-

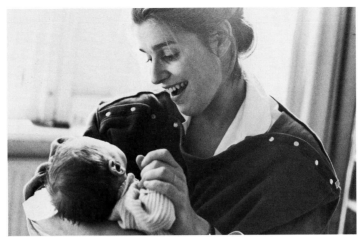

ing on myself. We arrived and checked in. Gauke said, 'We are going to the delivery room.' The man replied, 'Well, we shall call for you.' I felt like I was in a big department store or something. I disliked the hospital intensely. I was shoved into its system, and my situation and feelings faded in significance. The atmosphere of warmth and working together was gone, and the contractions almost stopped; they came every fifteen minutes, whereas before, they had come every three minutes.

We had rather bad luck with timing because there was an opening for a photographic exhibition in the hospital hall, and press photographers and lots of people were running around. We sat somewhat dazed. It took quite awhile before a student nurse found us. And when she did, she kept saying, 'I don't know what has to be done now.' My thought was, 'Help, what is in store for me?'

We went upstairs, and a very kind woman said, 'Please lie down.' When I said no, she said, 'You don't have to, of course.' I took off my shoes and walked around the room. They didn't quite know what to do with us. We stayed there for ten minutes, and in that time, three people came out and went without introducing themselves. Otherwise, nothing happened, and I continued doing what I had done at home, except now the interval between contractions lasted fifteen minutes. At a certain point, another person came in and said 'Come along', and we were taken into

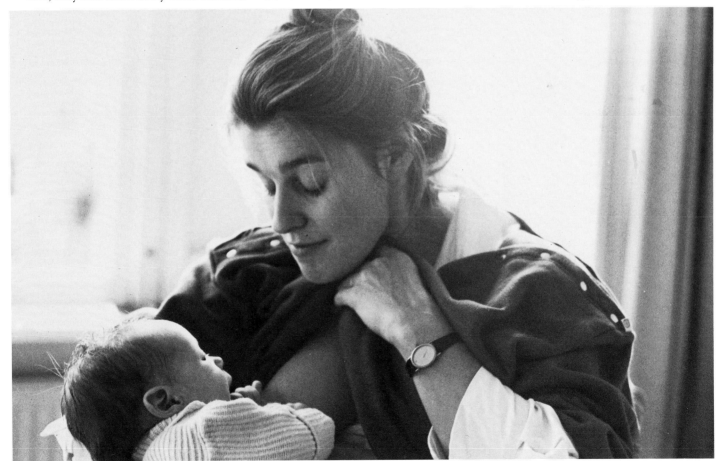

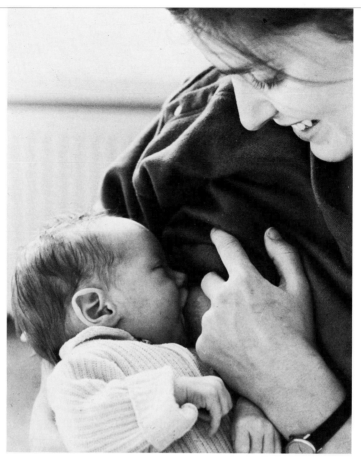

the delivery room, where we stayed. Henriette, a trainee midwife with whom I felt some sort of connection, stayed with us. 'We'd better lie down for a moment,' she said, 'so we can see how we are getting along.' The gynecologist found that I was dilatated six to seven centimeters. I had been pretty confused for an hour. After that, I was with it again and was able to take in everything—for instance, those stupid, gray bedside tables and that we had nowhere to hang our coats. Trivial things suddenly became very important.

Were there more important things about the hospital surroundings and procedures that disturbed you?

At first I wasn't pleased at the prospect of having lots of people present as I pushed out my child, but when it happened, I never really noticed them. That horrible strip lighting was awful but was necessary for the vaginal examination. I really disliked the apparatus with which they register the baby's heartbeat. They strapped two belts around my tummy—one for the heartbeat, and the other to measure the intrauterine pressure. Luckily, this didn't last long. Later, they screwed a little screw [internal monitor lead] into her bottom. They don't think about it. They learn it, they do it, and that is that. They even said, 'It isn't that we're suspicious....' I would have liked to have said, 'Do you know what you are doing, screwing a screw into her bottom? You don't even know for sure exactly where her bottom is.' This took place almost at the end. I really felt that my child couldn't handle

all this, having already worked so hard. Even now, Kyra still has a red mark on her bottom. But they told me it was necessary, and at that time I felt so helpless. I should have said, 'Don't do it, stop it, it's crazy, it's senseless! In other parts of the world, children are born without these things.' I simply didn't dare tell them what I thought. I also regret that I didn't stop them from putting silver nitrate drops in Kyra's eyes. I have to admit they did say, 'If you insist, we won't do it,' but I was unsure. I had read somewhere that it was not very good for the baby, and I thought it was an odd procedure, but because they said the doctor strongly recommended it, I thought it must be necessary. In retrospect, I feel that I should have never allowed them to do these things.

Did they explain to you why they felt the drops were necessary?

Yes, to prevent an eye infection that the baby may catch if the mother has gonorrhea.

Did dilatating those last centimeters take long?

Yes. At four o'clock I was dilatated seven centimeters, and Kyra was born at half past one. I think they examined me about 7:30 that evening, and I was still only eight centimeters. Everybody was disappointed. The contractions came every three minutes again. Beatrijs advised taking a shower. I shall be forever grateful to her for that suggestion. Doing something gave me the courage to go on.

At 11:30, I was about nine centimeters. At that point, I felt sort of intoxicated. During the vaginal examination, I realized that I must stay very close to my inner self and have the security of steady people around me. I think I could relax because I concentrated on each contraction. I felt them with my body, knew them in my head, and felt them in my heart. In ballet, there is a saying that the head, heart, and body are always in contact. The moment a contraction began, these three parts of myself merged, which helped me deal with the contraction until it passed. I felt very close to Gauke, and

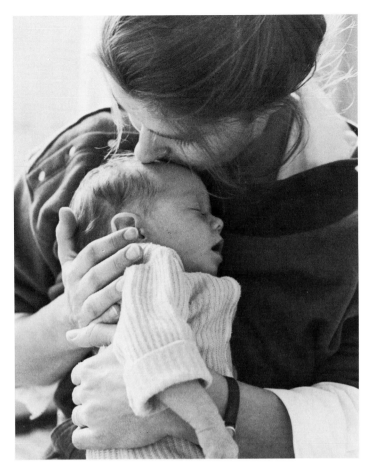

together we worked intensely. I wouldn't have been able to manage without Gauke, on whom I could hang and push, Henriette, and Beatrijs. I can still feel those three people around me, acting as a sort of rock.

You were given an infusion of synthetic oxytocin at the end of cervical dilatation. How did you feel about that?

It worried me. I don't really know what physical effects it had, but I couldn't find the courage to say that I didn't want it because I was in such a dependent position. They had examined me twice, and I was disappointed that I hadn't made any progress for hours. I remember thinking that they must help me because I can't stand this any longer, but if that had really been the case, I wouldn't have been able to even think that. If the baby had been lying normally, I might have said don't do it, but I knew that full dilatation of the cervix was vital because otherwise the baby could suffocate.

Did the contractions change after the infusion?

They became much more powerful and frequent. They came every other minute, so I was unable to walk. I sat on my bed and dangled my legs over the side. Henriette stood in front of me, and Gauke stood behind me. That small circle was everything—watching her and feeling him. Eventually, I felt very oppressed and felt I wouldn't be able to cope much longer. I was scared to death something might go wrong. The gynecologist came in again to examine me. I heard myself say that I couldn't stand it any longer. I was very conscious of the fact that I had lost control over my body and needed to push. She replied, 'Mothers usually can sense when it's time.' I was allowed to start pushing though I wasn't fully dilatated. Gauke and I hadn't prepared a specific plan for pushing. I searched for a comfortable position to push from, which took about five minutes. Then Beatrijs helped start to push.

While I was pushing, I had an almost Buddhist concentration. The pushing was painful. I seemed to have reached my limit—everything ached. Yet somehow I

knew exactly what I should do; otherwise I couldn't have managed. Everything came to us the moment we needed it. If I needed Gauke to lean against my right side, he would. I had to work harder and harder to concentrate so I'd be alert for the moment I needed to start breathing slowly. Gauke, who was breathing with me, would get out of rhythm, and I would take the initiative. Sometimes I would be too weak, and then he would guide me. Henriette helped me the whole time, and at the last stage of the pushing, I heard Beatrijs cry, 'Breathe in, breathe out now.' She seemed to be completely tuned in to me. There were rough moments, but also moments of perfect harmony, which are more interesting to remember than the pain. The pushing seemed to take only a minute, but, in fact, lasted twenty minutes.

What did you feel the moment you actually pushed out the baby?

Out of the corner of my eye, I saw Henriette putting a mirror underneath me. I did see Kyra's little bottom dangling, but I saw nothing else. I couldn't look anymore because I had to work from within. I felt as if an electric current went from my head through the middle of my body. This lasted for twenty minutes, but I can only remember the final moment, when she came out. I felt the exact contours of her body. That was wonderful. The buttocks were out already. I felt the widening of her belly, then more narrow, then broader at the shoulders, and felt the neck clearly. I had to persevere as I felt the head come out. I was very surprised when I saw pictures afterwards. She looked like such a round lump, but I really felt her as a series of shapes.

What was it like to see her for the first time?

I didn't feel she was my child, that is why surprise seems the most appropriate word. It was unreal to me that she was actually here. This feeling still overwhelms me now and then. I will never get over it in all my life. We were suddenly sitting on the floor; I have no idea how we got there. I saw her eyes before I'd seen she was a girl. I remember those eyes looking straight up. What is her name? someone asked. We hadn't been sure about a name, but at that moment it became very clear: Kyra. After that I simply enjoyed myself.

The first moments were very intense. What were your feelings in the days and weeks that followed?

From the beginning, the contact first thing in the morning has been the strangest. I felt spoiled that first week; everybody was very sweet. I felt my first real maternal instinct when she was ten days old. I went to the butcher shop, and they all came running to look at Kyra.

Did Gauke have trouble adjusting to the new situation?

Much more than me. I'll never forget how he looked when we came home. Gauke stood next to the bed he had made up so beautifully—he had gotten me flowers, too—looking like a ghost. He was dead tired for three days. Everybody came by to see Kyra and talk to me, and Gauke was left pouring the tea. He is also in the background in terms of contact with Kyra. At night, Gauke takes her out of her cradle and changes her diaper, but then she comes to me to be fed. In the beginning, she would return to him to cuddle or to burp, but I notice this is happening less.

I have got all the time in the world, whereas he has gone back to work.

Did you have any postpartum depression?

No, I didn't. Well, on the eighth day I did argue with Gauke. It was the last day the maternity nurse was going to be at the house. I was sitting on my bed, and when Gauke went off to work that afternoon, he said, 'I won't be home tomorrow evening, so let's see who can come and look after you and Kyra.' I burst into tears. I thought, 'This isn't possible. He wants to go away and leave me alone. I can't even walk properly yet and my tummy aches.' The maternity nurse left the room, which was tactful, and then I let go. I panicked and Gauke didn't understand my reaction. His attitude was that we could simply make arrangements. All that day I remained quite upset, but the next day was lots of fun again. And two days later, I really enjoyed being at home by myself.

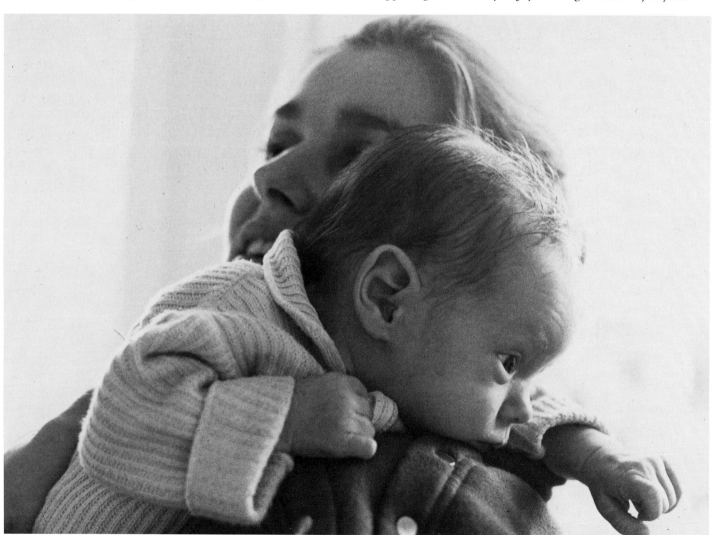

PART IV

First Contact with Your Child

Advantages of the Vertical Birth

T HE WHOLE DELIVERY is focused on how to get your child into the world, and then, suddenly, the child is here. In those first moments after the birth, feelings of surprise are stronger than any other emotion. You may experience childbirth just once or only a few times in your life, and its intensity is incomparable to anything else. Because the arrival of your baby can be overwhelming, it is advisable to go into the delivery with some idea about how you want the first contact with your child to proceed.

After the delivery, you will find that you need time to recover physically as well as to adjust to your child. It is important for the midwife to melt into the background, creating more space for the first encounter. In this initial orientation, both the parents and the child must assimilate brand new impressions.

If you remain vertical during and after the delivery, you are in a better position to participate in the astonishing emotional world of the first contact. You can watch your child being born onto a pillow or a soft piece of material. You stay in touch with yourself and the baby: you follow your own rhythm, your own feelings; you watch, touch, relax, and take the baby into your arms at the moment you and the baby are ready. Basically, no one else but you needs to touch the child. Being positioned vertically, you have control of such matters. Some women pick up their babies instantly, but most like to watch and touch the baby and become aware of their emotions before they hold their newborn. And processing feelings takes time. Frederick Leboyer, French obstetrician and author of *Birth Without Violence*, recommends massaging the child firmly for the first minutes after the delivery until it relaxes. If a mother is sitting up, she will be more inclined to do this because she is more active.

Once you have more or less recovered physically, you and your child can adjust to each other gradually. The vertical delivery facilitates this process; in an erect position, you are face to face with your child. The urge for contact is felt strongly by the baby. In a supine delivery, the child really exerts itself to turn and even lift its head toward the mother as she talks, an almost impossible task for a child lying on his or her mother's chest. A woman who lies on her back with her baby on her chest complains, "I can't see my child at all." Apparently, merely touching is not enough. Both mother and child have a strong yearning to see each other. The newborn needs time to adjust to much more light than he or she has been used to. This does not mean that a baby must be born in semidarkness; after all, plenty of children come into this world in bright daylight. It makes sense for the room to be lit sufficiently because the baby needs to learn how to see and could not see clearly in a dark room. Once the baby has acclimatized to its new surrounding, he or she will tune in to you. When you talk, his or her face will move toward the direction of your voice. At first the baby will look at you only momentarily, but each time the gaze will become longer. It may happen that your newborn looks at you alertly, as if he or she recognizes you.

The room where the baby is born need not be absolutely quiet as Leboyer advocates. A baby knows its mother's voice long before birth and is more or less familiar with the father's voice and the voices of others in the household. Most likely, sudden silence or whispering would seem odd to the baby. On the other hand, when Leboyer speaks about hospital deliveries, where the noise of an air conditioner or the impersonal voice of a stranger would be unfamiliar and confusing to the baby, his concern is justified. In a place with unfamiliar sounds, it is especially important that the baby can orient itself to the familiar voices of mother and father.

The room should be kept warm so mother and child can remain unclothed without becoming chilled. The baby can snuggle in its mother's arms and experience for the first time the warmth and smell of bodily contact. This often reassures and relaxes the child, who, nevertheless, often continues to whine or cry because he or she has become so excited.

Some children are so distraught from the birth efforts that they remain restless and tearful for quite some time. Often, they are able to relax in a warm bath, after which they are ready for all the new stimuli. In the Dutch home delivery, either the midwife, the maternity nurse, or increasingly often, the father bathes the child. If the woman is sitting, she can let the baby float in a tiny bath positioned between her legs. When the umbilical cord is long enough, she can even bathe her baby while he or she is still connected to her.

The aim of the bath is not to wash the child but to let the baby float and relax in warm water. Mother and father can bathe the baby together so the child is held by four hands. Another possibility with a home delivery is to take a bath with your baby. If you have a tub that is large enough, your partner can join you and baby in the water. Many babies are drawn very strongly toward their fathers. Sometimes the first contact with the father is more intense than that with the mother because she is often exhausted from giving birth.

Some women put the child to their breast instantly. The first powerful sucking movements usually occur a quarter to half an hour after the infant is picked up by the mother. The baby has to cope with many new stimuli and is often not ready to concentrate on sucking properly. The signals that indicate a child's readiness to suck are sucking movements of the mouth and tongue, lively hands, and half-closed eyes. When you see these, the moment to take your child to the breast has arrived. Holding the baby while sitting straight puts the newborn in an excellent position to search for the nipple. A baby explores the breast not only with mouth and tongue, but with hands and even feet.

About an hour and a half after the delivery, the baby will start to get tired and become distracted. This is the time to end the first encounter; during the days and weeks to come, you will have many opportunities to deepen your exploration of each other.

The first weeks after the delivery are tiring. Everything happens at once and everything is new. The days pass swiftly, you sleep little, and you have to develop a new rhythm. Friends and relatives come to visit you and the baby, which can be pleasant but very hectic. Stand up for yourself and your child during this period. In these first few weeks, the child needs every bit of time that he or she is awake to get acquainted with you. Your maternity nurse, partner, or other individual who is assisting you in this time of life transition will help you make arrangements so you give priority to your needs and those of the baby. Visitors can wait, you and the baby can't.

The photographs and interviews in this section portray the parents' experience of the initial orientation phase.

ELS AND MARC

Els: Merel's mother
Jeroen: first child, four-year-old boy (born in hospital)
Merel: second child, a girl (born at home)
Marc: Merel's father
Agaath: midwife

THIS INTERVIEW TOOK PLACE THREE WEEKS AFTER MEREL'S BIRTH.

When I visited you a week after the delivery, you told me that you were still very engrossed by it, that you dreamed about it a lot and were still mulling it over.

ELS: Every night at one o'clock, I used to get out of bed to write down everything that was turning over in my head and keeping me from falling asleep. Now, three weeks later, I am starting to relax. Giving birth is such a transition. Before the delivery I waited, unable to do anything; then, suddenly the baby takes up my entire day. My body changed abruptly as well.

I'm not sure whether this has anything to do with anything, but both Jeroen and Merel were born midsummer during a thunderstorm and at full moon. The days prior to and following the births were very beautiful. When Merel was born, our neighbor was being beaten by her husband. All the people we called were awake because of the storm. A girlfriend had had a dream in which I was delivering in the middle of the living room, though she was unaware that I intended to give birth there.

Do you consider birth violent?

ELS: It must be an incredibly violent event, for the child more so than for me.

MARC: Yes, Els and I talked about this a few days ago. Jeroen used to wake up at the exact time of his birth.

ELS: He would be awfully upset for about an hour. He suffered some sort of birth trauma and really needed to be comforted. Merel did not go through that.

What kind of experience was Jeroen's birth?

ELS: I was exhausted. I had not slept for three nights, and, of course, I was new at this and ignorant of what was awaiting me. The waters had broken and the contractions were not very strong. I was nervous because each time I thought it had started and then nothing happened.

We had been puttering around the house the whole night. We had gotten the bed ready and called the midwife who said she would pop by the next day, which was hardly reassuring. Twenty-four hours later, I had to go to the hospital because of the increased danger of infection. They immediately wanted to induce labor, but I told them I preferred natural birth, and, so after a lot of effort, I talked them into postponing it. Half an hour later, the contractions started on their own. It was totally different from my second delivery. I had to lie in bed and was not allowed to walk around. It hurt tremendously, and I couldn't control the pain. I noticed that this time around, too, the moment I lay down, I was in much more pain.

Lying down was awful?

My back ached horribly, preventing me from doing anything at all. During my recent delivery, I was talking and laughing between contractions. I was in control the whole time. During the hospital delivery, I didn't say a word because the pain would have driven me totally mad.

What else was different this time?

This delivery, I did much more myself and needed Marc's help much less. With Jeroen, I didn't want Marc to leave the room for a single second, and when he needed to, a nurse had to hold my hand, otherwise I felt totally lost.

I was more rested this time, and I was very active during the pregnancy. With a two-year-old around the house, you are running about and cycling all day long anyway.

MARC: We prepared ourselves differently this time. *New Life,* a book written by Janet Balaskas, helped us quite a bit. It showed squatting and stretching exercises.

Did you do squatting exercises?

ELS: Squatting comes naturally to me. The first time I exercised for a few minutes, and each time after that, a little longer. I also practiced kneeling on the ground with my bottom on the floor. This was impossible at first, but become easier when I did it regularly.

MARC: It was rather nice to have chosen and practiced a particular way of delivering—Michel Odent's supported squatting position.

You sat in a bath. Was that enjoyable?

ELS: Water alleviates a lot of the pain. The pain made me cranky. The moment I sank into the tub, I enjoyed the warm water and it relieved the pain. Still, I was drawn inward more and more. In between the first contractions, I was able to talk. I was still involved in the world around me. During the later ones, however, I con-

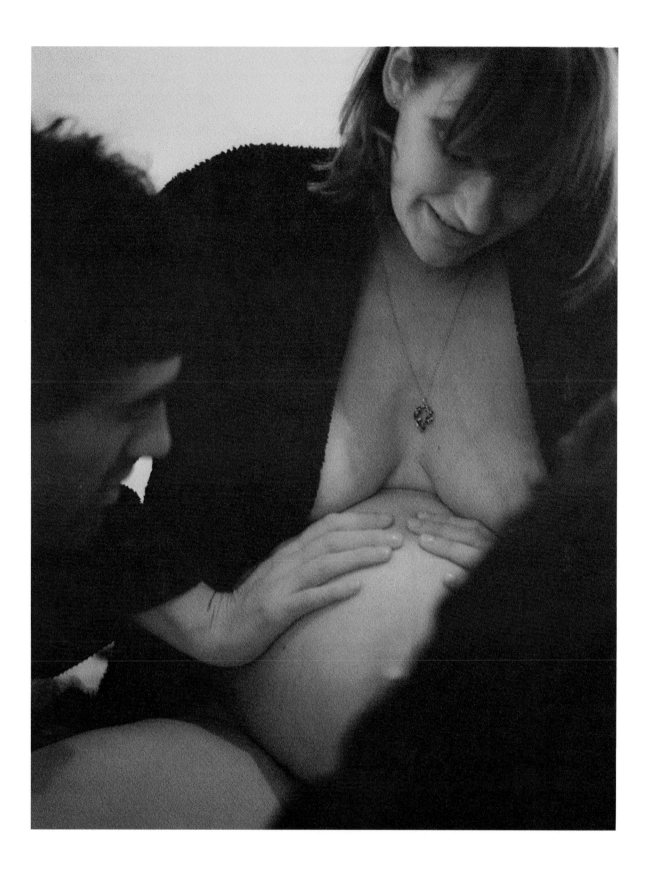

centrated solely on the delivery itself and could only do this with my eyes closed. Something happened to my body that I could not control. You can cry and scream as much as you like, saying you don't want it, but the more you resist, the more intolerable the pain. Your mind can either protest or cooperate. When Agaath announced the approach of the head, this dilemma disappeared because I again became fully aware of what I had been working toward. Marc was behind me and whispered, 'Stay close to your child.' I closed my eyes and was all right.

At a certain point, Agaath produced the mirror. Did you look into it?

I saw the head presenting itself, but then I shut my eyes. Handling what was happening outside as well as inside of me was too much. It distracted me. It did encourage me, though, because I knew the end was in sight. When Agaath pushed a small rim of my cervix over the baby's head, I was in great pain, but after that, things proceeded by themselves. I did not push, but only sighed, and the baby slid downward.

During the delivery, Els concentrated on keeping in contact with the baby inside of her. She talked to it quietly and used her hands to help the baby find its way through the birth canal. You and Marc practiced haptonomy, exercises to establish contact with the baby, from the fifth month of pregnancy on. An unborn child of that age reacts to stimuli from the outside world. By feeling the baby's movements, one can interpret these reactions. Did you get to know the baby a bit before it was born?

ELS: Touching your own tummy to feel your child is totally different from being examined by a midwife who searches for the baby with her hands. The medical examination is technical, checking the baby's size and position. When you put your own warm hand on your belly, it is intimate—that is really feeling! You ask for contact, you invite your child to come to you, you appeal to your child and it

recognizes that. It is a superb experience when it snuggles down into your hands.

When the child is awake, you can play with it, letting it rock in your hands. You attune yourself to that tiny individual in your tummy. I rocked Merel just after she was born in the same way while she floated in a little tub filled with warm water.

Marc, you are very interested in haptonomy and had contact with Merel and Jeroen before they were born.

MARC: Toward the end of Els's second pregnancy, Merel reacted strongly to our voices. She could differentiate them from the voices of strangers. When she heard unfamiliar voices while I was rocking her in my hands, she would stop moving as if scared. She would be as still as a statue.

Did you recognize them after the birth?

MARC: Jeroen was typically Jeroen: active, restless, reacting to the outside world, and extroverted. Merel is as calm now as she was in Els's tummy. She is much quieter than Jeroen and so I could not really register her reactions. She is so beautiful; her eyes radiate tranquility. Although you are in touch with your unborn child through haptonomy, the moment you actually see your child remains the most important. I could not experience entirely what was happening in Els's belly the way she could. That is simply impossible. I never knew that a woman draws into herself so deeply and that a man cannot empathize with her.

ELS: When I was pregnant with Jeroen, I was often cross and offended that Marc felt so little empathy with me. I understand better now why that was so.

You often hear about couple with young children getting divorced. This isn't strange. We went through rough times after Jeroen was born. It is much better now. The troubles started when I was pregnant with Jeroen. We could not agree on who would work and who would stay

at home. We agreed that we would share household and baby tasks equally, which proved to be unrealistic.

Jeroen's delivery mortified me and was the loneliest experience I have ever had. I felt lonely partly, I think, because I was so passive. Others directed the event; I simply endured it because I assumed that was how things ought to be done. I was not lonely at all during Merel's birth. I was in my own home among my own surroundings. I felt independent and was walking around. I was the one deciding what would happen.

Marc was very involved in the whole birth. He sat behind me to support me while I squatted, and when Merel arrived, he was fully present, which was fantastic. I picked her up immediately and pressed her to me. It was a continuation of the birth itself. For a moment, the outside world ceased to exist. It is an extremely intense moment, an awe-inspiring event. It is a curious mixture for the senses: the baby is warm, smooth, soft and has such a particular smell when it has just come from your tummy. Everything is so strangely familiar. You and your child approach each other, you touch and look, search and explore each other.

Has the experience of giving birth changed you drastically?

ELS: I feel more united with all living things. I have become part of the whole and am no longer merely an individual. To take responsibility for these young lives, a new generation, is a new experience. Life has a pattern of birth, life, and death—undulating motion—and my position on that wave has changed by having had two children. It has influenced my whole being and changed my vision of life. It has revealed to me the relationship between being young and growing older. I am more conscious of feeling that the duty of life on Earth is to provide a dignified existence for everybody. We must keep the world habitable for the generations to come.

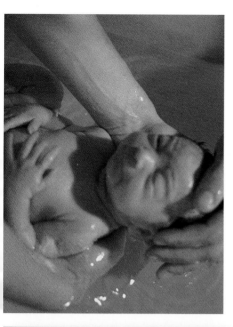

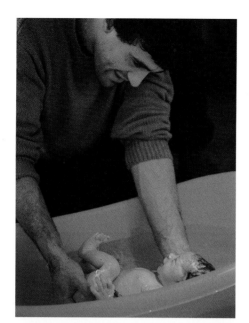

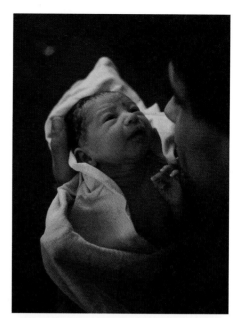

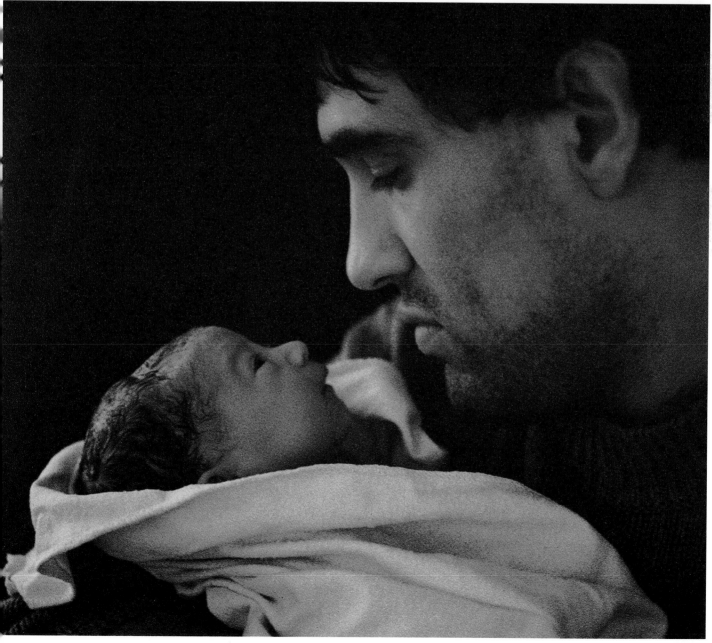

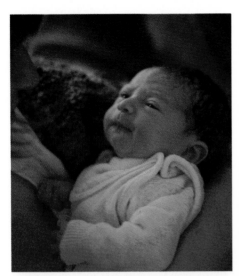
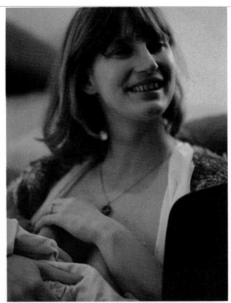
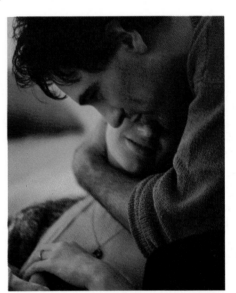
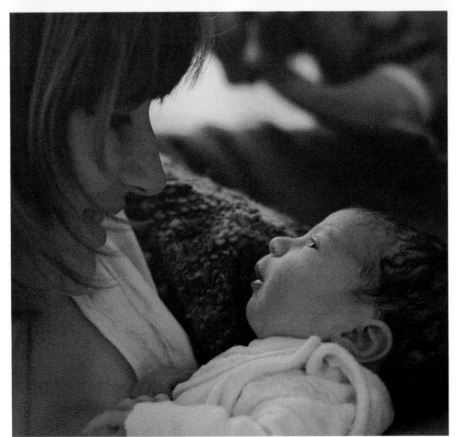
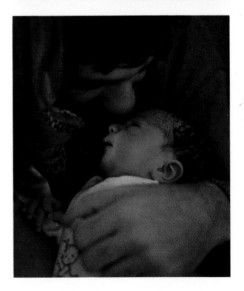

Margreet: Floortje's mother
Floortje: first child, a girl (born in hospital)
Martine: Margreet's aunt
Agaath: midwife

How did you choose who would attend the delivery?

It was obvious to me. They were girl-friends of mine, my aunt, and my mother whom I think of as a girlfriend. Their presence brought me a sense of security.

Had you consulted the hospital staff in advance about their presence in the delivery room?

No, because we actually had not planned it that way. I thought only my mother would stay with me, while the others would wait outside in the corridor. But the event ran its own course. It was grand; everyone was just transposed from one room to another.

Do you have a good relationship with your mother?

I've discussed many things with her; for instance, the fact that my father ob-jected to me having a baby. But in the end, he was so nervous, the way only a father can be, and very moved and sym-pathetic. He said some reassuring words at the last moment. My mother said it horrified her to see her child in pain. Now I know what she meant.

Did it remind her of her own delivery?

No, she did not think about it at the time. She was totally dedicated, which was lovely, and when, at times, she could not handle it emotionally, someone else took over for awhile until she had recovered and could continue to support me.

When the contractions started, she was awfully nervous, and I knew I first had to reassure her. She was ill at ease at the beginning because I was having diffi-culty breathing properly. Then Martine, who remains calm in any disaster, prac-ticed the breathing with me. From that moment on, my mother lost her anxiety.

When I arrived today, you were taking a bath and listening to beautiful music.

Vivaldi's *Four Seasons* is my favorite music. I craved that music because it has a soothing effect on me. I used to play it during my pregnancy when I felt like re-laxing or reading quietly. It does not evoke emotions that are too intense.

Did Floortje react to that music when she was inside you?

She did not react to that music, but I often attended concerts and she re-sponded then. She used to kick ferociously at the sound of modern music and be-came very tranquil when the music was peaceful.

As if she was listening?

Yes. I am convinced that babies can hear sounds before they are born, not as clearly as we perceive them, and they do respond. I often played the piano with my niece, and I am convinced that sooner or later Floortje will recognize that music.

Do you play for her these days?

I do not play a lot right now, but I play plenty of albums. She like that. I vis-ited my parents recently. My father sug-gested that my mother and I go shopping downtown while he took care of the baby. At one point, she started to cry, and he sat down behind the grand piano and im-provised music for her.

Have you ever been present at someone else's delivery?

Yes, I worked in a delivery room and witnessed approximately twenty deliver-ies. I was only seventeen years old, and I used to come into the room just in time to catch the baby. I had to bathe and dress the baby quickly. Then, it was given a medical examination, after which it either would be put in to a cradle or given back to the mother. It was a cold business, like a kind of sausage machine.

I imagine that such an experience does not leave fond memories. I was scared deliveries would be like that in every hospital.

Did your experience differ from what you had seen before?

Yes, I really felt that it was my deliv-ery. I indicated what I wanted and it hap-pened. This was absolutely unheard of ten years ago when the midwife, doctor, or nurse determined the course of things. In-variably, it was a panicky situation.

What was it like when labor actually started?

I hadn't an inkling of what a delivery actually entailed and hadn't really pictured it in my mind. I thought I would just go into it like that. The first contractions frightened me, and I panicked not know-ing where to sit or stand. It was the middle of the night and I worried about waking up everybody, so I decided to cope by myself as long as possible. I felt as if I was sitting in a cupboard, concentrating solely on these contractions. The things around me did not count anymore. I never wondered how long this would go on. It was timeless. I totally surrendered to nature. I could not control it anyway, so I thought I'd just take it as it came.

Did you feel that these contractions were serving a purpose?

No. I felt the pain, which excluded me from the world around me. I took things as they came. Being able to do that gave me a genuinely quiet feeling.

Although the contractions made you draw into yourself, do you feel you shared the experience of birth with the people who were in the delivery room?

At the time, I had tremendous longing for someone to be close to me. I needed contact. My relationships with the people who were present have deepened. We have shared something beautiful, something unique.

Some things escaped my notice or have slipped from my memory, like things I said at some point. I can talk with those who were there and everything comes back again. I really enjoyed having everybody there.

How was the experience of being pregnant?

It was difficult for me in the beginning. The first three months I reflected a lot. I had made a conscious decision to become pregnant, but, nevertheless, I thought about all the pros and cons. I expected people to react strangely, which used up lots of energy. The place I work was not flourishing at that time; they were cutting back and I brought the news that I was pregnant! But after that, I had a pleasant time. Everybody was so interested. It was incredibly cozy.

What about the physical transition?

I never had morning sickness. Well, perhaps a day or two, but more likely that was caused by nerves rather than by the pregnancy itself. I was not overtired. Luckily, I could do everything just as I did before. I radiated the fact that I could face practically anything.

What is it like to be in touch with someone you can't actually see?

I had a vague idea of what she looked like, but no real picture of her in my mind. That's why I was so pleased that she reacted; when I lay down, she would start to kick. I felt it a lot, but it remained somewhat unreal. I felt a sense of responsibility, and I have never lived a healthier life than during that time.

What did you dream about during your pregnancy?

I dreamed of children, but not about the delivery. In these dreams, my behavior with babies was criticized, and I thought, 'I am sure I am not doing this properly.' After the delivery had taken place, I dreamed that someone congratulated me for having had a son. I replied 'It is not a boy. I have a baby daughter.' Then, I called the general practitioner who asked me to come by, and he told me my baby was neither a boy nor a girl. I decided in that case he or she could choose what they wanted to be later.

In another dream, my twelve-year-old brother suddenly turned into a baby. I was worried and had to look after him constantly. Then something happened, and I was gripped by panic—the typical worry of responsibility—which will never disappear again.

My baby dreams were always set in the countryside in the company of many family members. In one dream, the family was enjoying a meal. Grandmother was the boss of the family, and all of us were sitting around her. I had a baby and had to leave the table incessantly in order to look after her. An unhappily married uncle remarked to his wife, 'You shouldn't spend so much money.' I asked him, 'What difference does it make, she has a big hole in her hand?'

What kind of relationship did you have with your midwives?

I was anxious and apprehensive at the first meeting. Later we had discussions; it was pleasant to be able to ask them questions. I had heard of them and knew that all three were highly capable. I was familiar with their ideas and concepts of giving birth.

Did you discuss in advance whether you would deliver vertically?

I chose these midwives because I wanted to have a vertical delivery. I knew they used that method. I had heard on a radio program that such deliveries go smoothly and quickly.

In the end, you delivered vertically, without a bed, in a delivery room in a hospital.

Even at that moment I was afraid I wouldn't be able to squat, but it all went fine.

Had you practiced squatting during your pregnancy?

I had made a few attempts, but I couldn't do it.

But during the delivery it went perfectly all right?

Yes, I thought I would have to squat with my feet flat on the ground, but that is not how I did it. Assuming the squatting position seemed quite natural to me.

By 'squatting' do you mean the supported squatting position?

Yes, it struck me as the most natural position to deliver a child.

You tried out several positions during the period of cervical dilatation, didn't you?

Not deliberately; luckily, it just happened that way. I simply enjoyed alternating between sitting on my knees with my head bent to the ground and walking or looking out of the window.

Did those signals come from within?

Yes, and I obeyed them automatically. I was concentrating so hard on the pain that I did anything to help alleviate it a little.

At one point, I felt Agaath's hand on

my lower back; somehow this distracted me from the pain. I asked my mother to do the same. She did not massage me but simply put her hand there, which was relaxing.

Were you in touch with your child during the delivery or were you more involved with yourself?

My only worry was not to hurt her and not to get hurt myself. During the pushing, I was afraid I would tear despite the easy progress of the birth.

Did you feel her descending while you were pushing?

Yes, very distinctly. The farther the contractions pushed her down, the more fearful I became. Someone said that I was almost there, but I did not believe it. That is why I refused to look into the mirror.

Did you look into it in the end?

I looked at it once, but I did not want to spend my energy on that. Seeing what you are feeling at the same time you are feeling it can have the wrong effect.

How did you feel during the first moments after she had been born?

It was beautiful but unreal, I did not instantly feel, 'this is my child.' It is a human being on its own with whom I have to become acquainted. There is a tie, but it is without form yet. You should merely watch during those first moments. I did not check to see whether I had a boy or a girl. It was a human being and its sex was irrelevant to me.

Do you remember the moment you picked Floortje up?

I realized I had to be very careful because she had just gone through great difficulties. So many emotions were going through me at the same time.

You put her down for a moment and then picked her up again.

I did that partly because the umbilical cord was so short and partly because I wanted to look at her more.

Did you start to touch her then?

I wanted to feel her skin. The grease on her skin felt so smooth that I rubbed it in a bit. I was astounded. While she was still attached to me by the umbilical cord, I was convinced she was a boy.

Did she cry?

No, it surprised me that she hardly cried at all and started looking around instead, watching me especially, which she still does now.

Did you bathe her yourself?

I was sitting with the baby bath between my legs. The umbilical cord hadn't even been cut yet. It was rather short, but that didn't matter. She loved it. She was looking around in wonder and did not cry at all. She thought the water was blissful. I felt that nothing could go wrong because she was still attached to me.

You gazed at her endlessly, played with her, rocked her.

I had to explore everything about her. All her reactions were new, and it was splendid to see something of myself react. All of her reactions, to being bathed or to the people around her, surprised me.

Did she watch you, too?

Yes, she also looked at me with those inquisitive eyes.

Do you think she responded to you as you talked to her?

As soon as I started talking, she looked straight at me. Naturally, she was very familiar with my voice. She seems to hear no other voices. The moment I talk, she knows I am close and looks, searching for the origin of the sound.

When was the cord cut?

That took ages. I think the moment the placenta arrived. I am not exactly sure how long it took but quite a long time. When I put her to my breast and she started sucking, I could feel that the placenta was on its way. My mother cut the cord.

What did you think of the afterbirth?

It is something you have to get done. I have seen many placentas in my life but was curious to see my own. It was exciting to examine it carefully.

Did she suck immediately when you put her to your breast?

Not in the beginning. Her mind was distracted by other things. It took a little time before she really started to suck properly. It must be an incredible experience to move from the womb into a big space full of people. To my surprise, she did exactly as she pleased in spite of other people's expectations. For example, she clearly indicated, 'It is not time to eat yet; I have too many things to absorb and process.'

How did you recognize when she was ready to eat?

I believe Agaath suggested I should try again. It took some time getting used to. I have assisted other mothers with putting their babies to the breast, but I felt uncertain about it with my own child. It went much better the second time, and she was suckling away to her heart's content.

How was getting up for the first time after the birth?

I felt as if I couldn't get up by myself, as if someone had kicked hard against my tailbone. Once I was up, I was pleasantly surprised that I could manage by myself, and that I could take a shower on my own.

After all the initial emotions had passed, I was left with a rather empty feeling. There was so much food for thought, but I could not deal with everything at that moment.

What I liked best was lying in the room with her, feeling my child in my arms, watching her. At a certain point, I was getting tired and fell half asleep; I noticed she was doing the same. I thought that she must feel the same way I did. I was still in sync with my child. I recognized myself in certain facial expressions, even though I had never really seen them in my own face, and felt our connection very strongly.

A living mirror so to speak?

Yes, it is amazing. I believe all mothers find this to a certain extent.

Do you look at her a lot?

Yes, especially at her expressions. At times when I am breastfeeding her and talking to her at the same time, I become unaware that I am feeding her, and it seems she feels totally the same way. When she is cross, she throws me angry looks with the same dark, flaming eyes that I have.

Does she look around a lot?

As soon as she wakes up, her eyes search the whole room. She follows every sound with her eyes. She can be really amused by something she sees. Floortje even laughs at her own noises. She finds sneezing hysterically funny.

During the first weeks you had to get used to breastfeeding. How did that go?

In the beginning, I clung to other people's opinions on breastfeeding because I was inexperienced. Then I realized that their ideas did not work for me. The first week was difficult, partly because I was tense. I had hoped to find peace in the hospital, but I felt quite the opposite. The stress reduced the amount of milk I produced. I had always believed that I wouldn't have any problems breastfeeding my baby. That first week was a disaster.

Did things pick up after you returned home?

All the guests who came to meet the baby affected the breastfeeding. I was worried that she might not get enough so I responded to people absentmindedly. I could not breastfeed her when other people were present. It was a matter of self-confidence.

What do you think of night feeding?

Now, I feed her for the last time at midnight, but I used to enjoy the night feedings. I'd take her into bed with me, and both of us would fall asleep until the next morning. It was very cozy. At first I was bothered because I thought this wasn't done, but later I read that it is fine. A baby never rolls out of bed because it is always drawn to its mother and will search for the breast when it is hungry. Since then, I haven't worried about this anymore. She is fine as long as she is at my side. She is comfortable so she doesn't cry.

It's hard to divide yourself in two, isn't it?

I am trying to do that all the time. There is something new in my life that I have to adapt to, but, at the same time, I must begin my social life again.

How fast does life begin to get back to normal?

Very slowly. Only now do I feel that I can distance myself from my worries about her. In the beginning, I hardly dared to leave her to run to the bank. I was rushing around. I could not relax even though a babysitter was looking after my child. When I went shopping, I would break into a cold sweat and race through the shop. Things are better now as long as I know that a responsible person is at home with her.

Do you feel that your view of life is changing

I come second now. I went away for a few days; normally I would take a big bag of clothes for myself. Now it is more important that her things are packed.

Had you expected that you would be like that?

No I hadn't. I have to prevent myself from talking endlessly about the baby. I am paying more attention to what other people are thinking because one day she might share their beliefs.

I have a beautiful book by Carl Jung that deals with the child archetype. The child is endowed with a pure soul that absorbs everything around it, including the mother's influence. She is still so pure and taking in so much.

MIEKE

I grasped Tim to help him come out of me. I was startled that he felt so slippery. He came out just like that. Indescribable, blissful. Everything was over and the only thing left was Tim.

I had not thought about what he would look like. I had been more concerned that he get to know Frans and me so he wouldn't feel like a stranger in this world. After all, it is not easy to be brought into this world like that, with no way back and no choice but to enjoy it. I know Tim recognized our voices because we used to talk to him every night when he was still in the womb. He would listen and hear it all. He seemed entirely happy lying with me, feeling secure while he slowly got acquainted with his new surroundings. He knew my heartbeat and could cling to that familiar sound. I really believe that is why he stopped crying immediately.

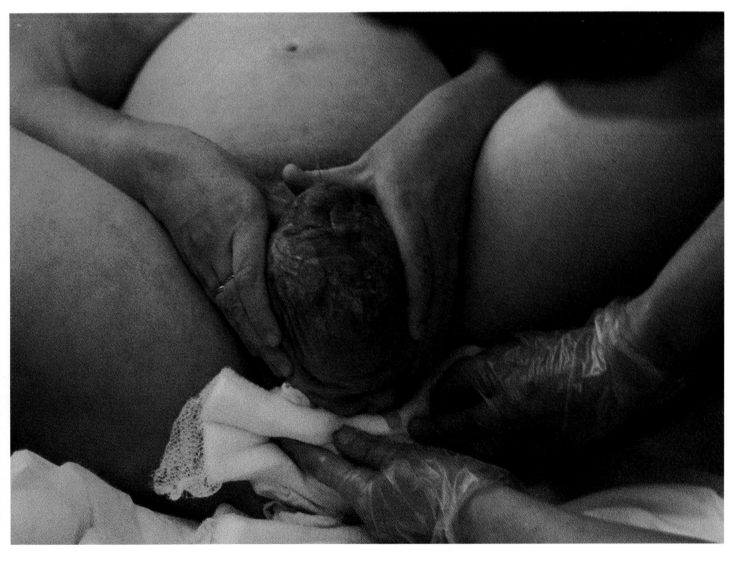

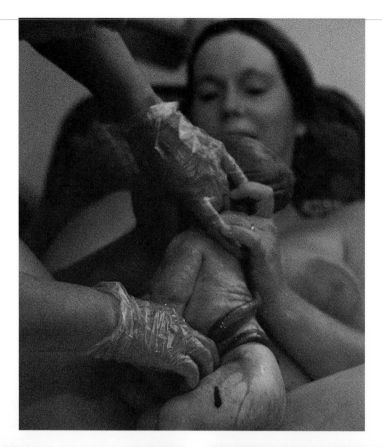

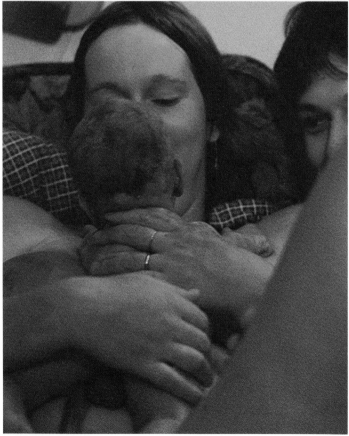

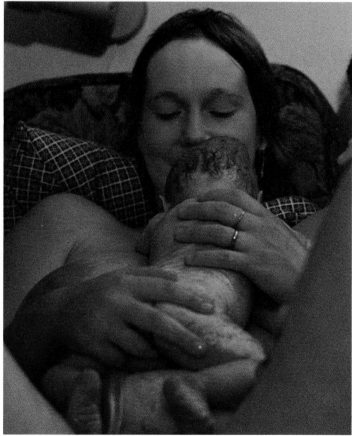

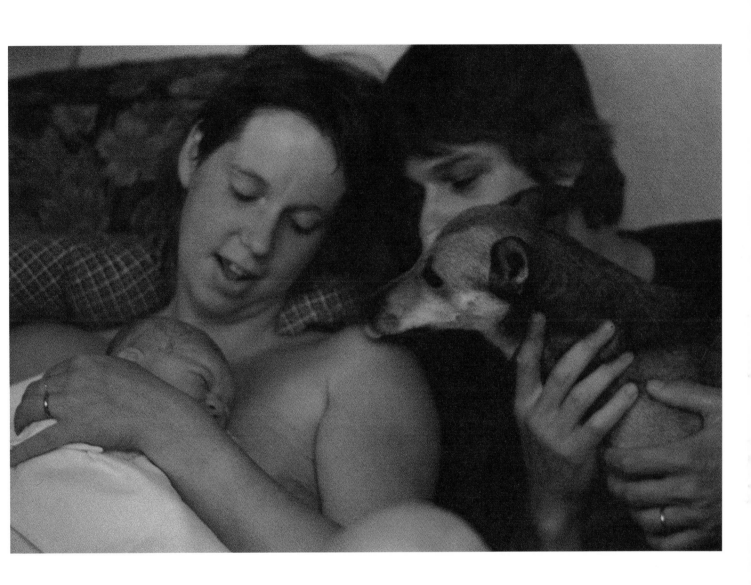

INGRID

Ingrid: Nina Liza's mother
Nina Liza: first child, a girl (born at home)
Hiep: Nina Liza's father
Agaath: midwife

THIS INTERVIEW TOOK PLACE SEVEN WEEKS AFTER NINA LIZA'S BIRTH.

You had asked your mother to be at the birth. What did her presence mean to you?

INGRID: She is someone who can tackle anything in any situation, so her presence was reassuring to me. She was a little anxious, but I was absolutely determined to have her there to experience the delivery.

Did she help you cope with the contractions?

That happened spontaneously. My mother gave birth to several children, so I knew she would be able to support me in this. Hiep had started to massage me but was not very good at it. My mother took over at her own initiative. Although she has never practiced massaging, she was great. A woman senses more accurately what you need.

I suppose that being Belgian she only had experience with hospital deliveries.

Yes, the people I know from Belgium are incredulous that I delivered in my home in Amsterdam without any injections and instruments.

How did your mother feel about your decision to give birth at home?

In the beginning she was anxious, and at the end she was amazed. In her mind, a delivery could only take place in a hospital. Her first delivery was extremely difficult whereas Nina Liza came out just like that. She could not believe I could muster the strength to shower afterwards and play

with the baby as well. That was completely new to her.

Do you have a different relationship with you mother now?

In a way, I feel we have experienced something beautiful together, but we don't put it into words. I sense that she is proud to have been able to experience her granddaughter's birth.

During the cervical dilatation contractions you played wonderful Greek music. You even danced to it. Tell me about that.

I had read you could do anything you felt like doing, and I relax best when listening to music and dancing. I did that during the pregnancy, too. The music reminded me of my vacations in Greece; listening to it, I saw the mountains and the colors and smelt its scents. I could feel that warmth.

You delivered in the living room. Is that where you had imagined the birth would take place?

I intended to deliver in the bedroom, but there was not enough space. I would have felt claustrophobic and wouldn't have been able to do much. In the living room I could move around, walk into the kitchen, listen to music, look outside and watch the boats sailing by—all these things are pleasantly distracting.

Had you dreaded the contractions?

No, I knew my body was meant to cope with them. I was curious about what would happen, which gave me a strong incentive to cope adequately. The con-

tractions started at night. I became restless and wondered whether to call the midwife. I went to the bathroom often. I attempted, without success, to fall asleep again. As dawn drew closer, I had quieted down somewhat.

Can you share the birth process with someone else, or is it a private experience?

The latter. I tried to share it, but I had difficulty putting it into words. The further into the delivery, the less conscious I was of the outside world. At first, I still felt involved in the outside world, but toward the end I certainly did not.

Were the contractions the reason you drew into yourself?

I believe so. They claim your attention; you have to concentrate all the time. Perhaps other women are able to share this, but Hiep was too upset and restless.

Did you take a prenatal class, and did it help you in any way?

Yes. During the pregnancy, it reassured me. I was able to talk with others about being pregnant and to reflect on my feelings and experiences. Having had the class was not of much help to me during the actual delivery. During the contractions, I did apply some of the techniques that I had learned, but most of the time, I just let them come and improvised. In a situation like giving birth, it is silly to stick to rules.

Were you sick during the first trimester of your pregnancy?

I was hopelessly sick, and for three months I could hardly get up in the morning. As the months passed, I felt better. In the beginning, I kept on running to the bathroom to vomit. I laid in bed for days on end. Going out was precious though. You carry your child in you and you both go out. When I stopped for a cup of tea, I always had company. I turned inside myself and lived in a dream.

Does morning sickness prevent you from having a positive feeling about your baby?

No, I was willing to sacrifice feeling good for a while in order to have a baby. I had been given some homeopathic pills, but I hardly ever touched them. The first part of my pregnancy was in the winter so I was indoors a lot, which I think made me feel even more sick.

What type of connection do you have with a baby you can't see yet?

I was burning with curiosity and kept touching my tummy to feel something move. I read plenty of books, and by looking at photographs of each stage of a baby's development, I could picture what I was carrying inside me at that particular time. This is how I kept in touch with her.

When did you first feel her move?

That happened quite early, in the fifteenth week. The midwife claimed that it was impossible, but I felt her as a butterfly fluttering in my belly, a slight vibration. I dreamed a lot those first few months. That subsided later when we were rebuilding and redecorating our houseboat. But toward the end, the dreams came back.

Did you dream about the delivery?

Once, I dreamed that the baby was born almost without effort. I felt great relief that it was over. Another time, I dreamed I gave birth to a child without a head. I had always had a hard time locating the baby's head. I could feel its arms, back, bottom, and its feet, but the head was situated too deeply in my belly.

Was she active during your pregnancy?

She was moving all the time, which made me expect a hot-tempered child. In reality, she is a rather quiet girl. I would stroke her back and try to get a hold of her feet.

During the cervical dilatation contractions you tried out several positions. Which ones did you like?

At first, I hung onto Hiep's neck, but as the delivery progressed, that position was no longer enjoyable. Sitting on a chair was comfortable, but being in the bath was heaven! It must be ideal to deliver underwater because the water carries your weight; unfortunately, our bath was too small for that. Walking around was also pleasant, but the most important thing was that someone was with me to support me as I had a contraction.

Did you have to push for a long time?

I pushed very little, perhaps two or three times. Pushing happens by itself; you need not do anything yourself. In fact, I had to resist pushing. I kept thinking, 'I must pant!' I was afraid of perineal tears. It was over before I knew it. That moment was totally overpowering. I was overwhelmed and had no idea what was happening.

Did you feel Nina Liza emerge from you?

I remember that sensation very clearly, and I never want to forget it. It was glorious—warm and slippery. I felt the arms and legs come out of me, and the umbilical cord. It was warmer than I was.

What were your impressions the first time you saw her?

Her face was surprising. She was a completely unique human being. She moved and uttered sounds, and she came out of my own belly. When I was pregnant, I had often felt her arms and legs moving around busily, and she was active in that same way after she was born. But the little face: the nose, the eyes, and its expressions were so amazing. And the way she cried, and the fact that sounds were coming from her throat.

Did you watch her for a little while before you picked her up?

Yes, I was absolutely stunned that a human being was lying there as if from out of the blue. When I touched her, I knew she was not as delicate as I had imagined, so I held her.

Hiep sang for her immediately, didn't he?

We had chosen her name from an Italian song we both love. Because he had sung it often during the pregnancy, Hiep felt like singing to her at that moment to express his emotions. We had read that unborn babies can hear sounds, so perhaps she recognized Hiep's voice at the birth. Now, we often perform for her and can tell how much she enjoys that.

How did you feel about the afterbirth?

It was not important to me because I was sitting and holding my little baby. I liked seeing and feeling the placenta's velvety texture, but focusing on her was more important. She was watching me, looking a bit dazed. She was slightly bewildered by the light and all the movement. She was unaccustomed to physical contact with me, but she enjoyed the warmth of my body and was reassured by the hollow I formed with my arms.

Is Nina Liza awake much of the time?

Yes, and she looks around. I try to see the room through her eyes. I walk around with her to show her the whole house. Every day she makes a new movement from which I can tell what she wants. For example, she puts her hands into her mouth or pouts when she is hungry. One gesture still puzzles me—she keeps sticking out her tongue. At first, I thought this meant that she was hungry, but that is not it.

What sorts of sounds does Nina Liza make?

She sounds contented when she is eating, and she babbles to herself when she lies in her cradle looking around the room. At first, I assumed she wanted to be fed, but she is just making noises to her toys, as if she wants them to answer. She is fascinated by her little monkey and often looks at it. I think she believes that it is a human being. When I put her into her cradle against her will, I put the monkey next to her, she looks at it, and it keeps her quiet for a while.

Does Nina Liza have her own room?

She always sleeps in our bed. She has a cradle, but she is miserable when I put her in it. She lies there during the daytime, but at night she joins us in bed. It makes feeding easier. She is calm when she knows that I am next to her. When I wake up in the morning and look into that sweet little face, I am thrilled.

How does she react to visitors?

That depends on how awake she is. If she is awake, she will smile at some people, like my mother, but not at others.

How does a relationship with an infant differ from that with an adult?

Adults are independent. She needs me. She is so small, so sweet; she is new, and I can look after her. I am full of expectations. Each day I wonder what will happen. What's the next step? Will she recognize me?

Has birth affected your relationship with Hiep?

Yes, I am more involved with Nina Liza, and I pay less attention to him. At times, he feels a bit pushed into a corner, but he makes this clear to me and we discuss it.

When she cries, I must go to her. Hiep can wait, but the little one can't. He keeps very busy with his music, and I require less attention from him now. In the past, I always wanted him to spend as much time with me as possible, but now I let him go much more. I couldn't raise her on my own though. The thought alone makes me have weird dreams.

Do you want to go back to work yet?

No, I enjoy running the household, bathing and feeding her, and going out for walks with her.

Has she changed you?

Before, I was more involved with my own life; now, Nina Liza is the most important thing to me, and I am willing to sacrifice anything for her. Nowadays, I talk with people more. I used to be more introverted. Having a child makes me feel more grown up. What I enjoy most is sitting in a cozy nest with her, watching her and dreaming away. I have to be able to let go of her at times, but if I had it my way, I would tie her to my belly day and night. Perhaps this will pass as she grows older.

BETTINA

Bettina: Dominique's mother
Dominique: first child, a girl (born at home)
Geert: Bettina's boyfriend
Rieke: girlfriend
Astrid: midwife

THIS INTERVIEW TOOK PLACE FIVE WEEKS AFTER DOMINIQUE'S BIRTH.

Geert, what is it like for you not being the child's father?

GEERT: It is a long story. Bettina, how long have you talked about wanting to get pregnant?

BETTINA: I had been fairly determined for about a year. I have always wanted to have a child but had not decided when. I discussed my ideas about raising children with Geert a few years ago. I was not quite sure what I wanted. I was sure that I did not want to have a baby within the traditional family structure, me living with a husband and a child in one house. I was just as strongly opposed to the idea of living alone with my child in an apartment. In the end, everything has worked out the way I wanted. Basically, I am a single parent, but other people in this house feel involved with us and participate in our lives.

GEERT: We went over this again a year before Bettina got pregnant. It seemed like an excellent idea, and I was considered a potential father until I was offered the opportunity to live here. I had a choice: become the father or a housemate. I preferred the latter.

Who was strict about carrying out the plan?

GEERT: I was. I absolutely refused to combine the two roles. It would only complicate things more. It was apparent that Bettina wanted to raise the child on her own. This could only be done if the father did not live under the same roof.

What makes you think that?

BETTINA: I believe it is natural for the father to feel a strong connection to his child. I had told Geert that I wanted a child, but without the presence of a traditional father, and that I had thought of him as a possible means to this end. He felt that he would rather live with me and my child than to be the child's father and live elsewhere. I was pleased that he had given it a lot of thought.

GEERT: I mulled over the idea for two weeks. I wouldn't mind becoming a father. Then it occurred to me that I would much rather live with Bettina instead. She seemed like she would be a good mother—which has proved to be true—and that gave me confidence.

How does the natural father feel about this arrangement?

BETTINA: He is not very clear about this. When I told him I wanted to have a child, and wasn't using any form of birth control, he sort of left the decision to me. He said he would not mind having a child, but he did not want to be responsible for it—he didn't feel ready for that yet. But if I was set on having a baby, it was my choice, and he wouldn't stop me.

How did the other people you are close to, like your family and other housemates, react?

Bettina: It was not a surprise to any of the people I live with. Everybody is familiar with my views on childrearing. My parents were shocked that I did not want to get married. My mother's first remark after I announced that I was pregnant was

'Well, are you going to get married now?' It took her some time before she could accept it—in fact, until the baby was born—and my father still does not approve.

GEERT: My mother worries about the child's situation—alone, surrounded by so many adults. She is also concerned about whether Bettina will be able to cope on her own. Her worries are not entirely unfounded, because however much we help Bettina, in the end, she is the one who is responsible. We are not obliged to share a house with her for the rest of our lives, but she will be tied to her child for life.

How do you feel about this, Bettina?

BETTINA: So far, everything has been marvelous. I get more support from my housemates than I had ever imagined possible. I had not really worried about it. I had no specific expectations of people, but I knew there would be people to give me support before, during, and after the delivery. And that has been the case. Up to now, everything has gone very well, but I do not feel tied down in any way. If anything were to go wrong between all of us and I wanted to leave with my child, I am sure I would find another community that would suit my needs and personality. I feel confident that I will always be able to find, or to create, a situation in which I am not entirely on my own.

RIEKE: When Bettina told me she was pregnant, I considered having a child in the same manner: having a child as a single parent and raising it in a group. My

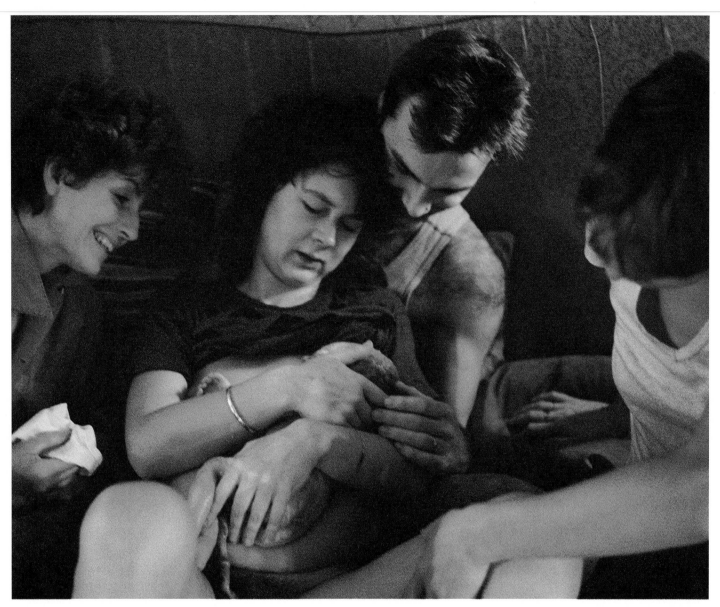

reaction to Bettina's pregnancy was that a child was on its way, and I might as well help raise and look after it. Like Geert, I do not feel that in order to participate it might necessarily be my own child.

GEERT: If anything happens to Bettina, someone will be granted custody of Dominique. The judge would ask all parties involved what Bettina would have wanted. If it becomes clear that Bettina intended Rieke to have custody, in general, Rieke would be allowed to take care of her. Dominique would not be placed with a traditional family. This is different from adoption. In such an event, I would be coguardian.

Perhaps I will want a child of my own ten years from now, or maybe sooner, but I am too restless now. I feel a sense of responsibility toward Bettina, which she feels toward me as well. We felt this for each other long before we started living together, and it will continue even if we live apart. I can't just drop people like that.

RIEKE: In your case, you two have built up a relationship over some time; I only met Bettina when I joined this household, so a different situation has developed between the two of us. When you live in a community, you feel closer to some people than to others. If something bothers me, I tend to go and see Bettina about it.

Had you always planned that the three of you would be at the birth?

GEERT: Rieke and I were excited about the idea of all three of us enrolling in the pregnancy course. We were sure it was something new.

BETTINA: We had come to a decision about both of them being at the birth when I was five months pregnant. In a Consciously Unmarried Mothers booklet, I had read about a woman who had asked two people to be with her during the delivery and had regretted it afterwards because she would have preferred to concentrate on only one person. But I like Geert and Rieke equally, felt I needed both of them, and thought there would be ample work for both of them.

RIEKE: It seemed like an excellent

idea to me, not only because it would be very tiring to support Bettina all alone, but because sharing the birth would keep this household balanced.

I was totally tuned into Bettina's needs: how was she feeling and what I could do for her. I benefited from the books I had read in preparation. We practiced some breathing techniques, but we concentrated most on relaxation. During the birth, this was achieved mainly through bodily contact.

BETTINA: The things they did spontaneously made it so pleasant. Rieke started massaging my legs, which was lovely. The same applies to the situation in the bathroom: I had not asked them to support me—Rieke initiated it—and it was very comfortable. They were full of ideas the whole time.

GEERT: I massaged her back until she wouldn't let anyone touch her. At that point, she hit me and cried, 'leave my back alone!'

Did you enjoy his touch in the beginning?

BETTINA: It was bliss to have my back massaged.

GEERT: Initially, she wanted us to touch her firmly. Later, she preferred to be touched more gently, and then she wanted only a hand there to support her. Finally, any touch was intolerable. After about three hours, we were not allowed to touch her belly or back.

Was the birth difficult for you? Had you practiced relaxation and breathing exercises?

BETTINA: I did exercises every night for six weeks straight. I had imagined the delivery would be totally different. I had counted on less pain. I had assumed— because I was so well informed and felt so self-confident and because I had carefully prepared myself for the delivery— that the pain wouldn't be so bad. I thought, 'I know how to relax so I will just do it in a couple of hours.' But it was tremendously painful.

RIEKE: You can never tell what a birth will be like, or how long it will last because each one is different in terms of its duration. Some women prefer to be active, and others like to be more passive. Bettina preferred to collapse completely. On our way to the bathroom she sank to the ground, and we held her.

Did you want to be active?

BETTINA: In the beginning, I felt like being active and climbed in and out of bed in order to get some exercise.

GEERT: For a long time, she would

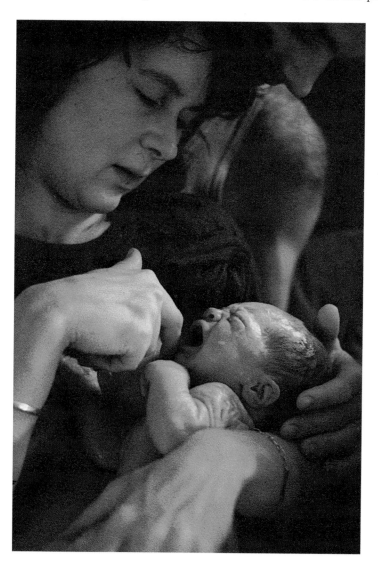

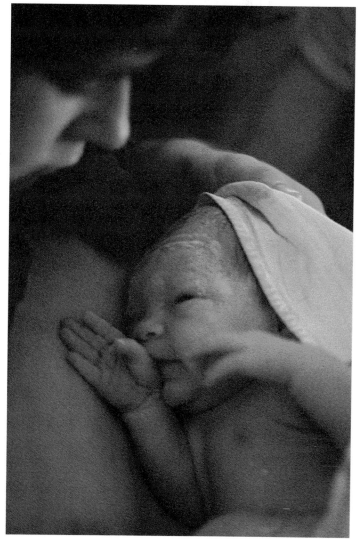

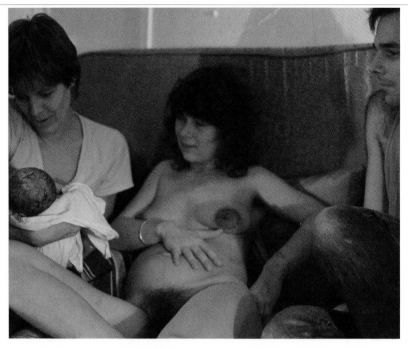

get out of bed, turn around, lean on the bed, kneeling down and hanging forward a bit. She could have used a chair, but apparently that did not work for Bettina.

BETTINA: If I moved at the beginning of a contraction, it didn't last as long. Later, however, I was unable to move at all.

Did you spend some time in the bath?

BETTINA: Yes, at two points during the delivery. I was yearning for a hot-water bottle or a hot bath. I loved sitting in the bath and being held under my arms by Geert and Rieke so I did not have to support myself. I didn't feel like lying down, so it was lovely to just lean on their arms without having to tense one muscle.

Did you mind the vaginal examination?

I did not mind at all because Astrid did it upon my request. She examined me three times. The first time, when she arrived, because I wanted to know how far I had dilatated, and she waited until I asked for the second exam. Just before I started to push, I asked her to examine me again because I was dying to start pushing.

What kind of relationship did you have with your midwives?

I like all three of them, but I would have preferred to have had a more personal approach. I was weak physically, and moody, too. In all those months, I was never really cheerful. I was hungry all day long, but I did not want to give in to hunger all the time. I woke up hungry at night, and I hated not being able to sleep through the night in one stretch. It frustrated me that I had to get up every night to eat something.

RIEKE: We discussed this with the midwife. Bettina was depressed and wasn't feeling well at all. The midwife explained that this was caused by hormonal changes, making Bettina more emotional than usual. It takes energy to deal with those emotions, so it was good to eat. Bettina resented eating and did not want to put on weight.

Did the three of you discuss this situation?

BETTINA: I hated myself for annoying everybody and for not being cheerful. I was worried all the time and suspicious of what people said.

GEERT: Bettina had a rough time, but things were not easy for me either. This has been the most difficult period of our friendship. I could not handle it, which disappointed me. On the other hand, I felt that Bettina was totally impossible to be with. She tired me out. There was lots of tension, which escalated into blazing rows.

We learned how to deal with it by talking to others. I think it taught us a lot, and now we are much closer because Bettina expressed more clearly what she wanted and let us know when she was feeling well so we could have fun together.

It is really important to be open about things and not to presume you understand each other because you have known the other person for a long time. It does not work that way.

Has your relationship changed since the birth?

GEERT: I was relieved that she became herself again. The evening after the delivery, her normal face returned. Our relationship is more intense now.

BETTINA: I was so overjoyed to see my figure return that I reacted to things the way I used to and was happy again. Besides, I felt fine in the final months of pregnancy.

RIEKE: When the prenatal course began, the three of us attended and had something to work towards together.

BETTINA: This coincided with my life finally being in order. I had passed my last examinations. I had planned on indulging myself and having fun for six weeks while I got well rested for the delivery. And I did.

GEERT: The delivery was the focus of our lives. Every night we exercised the pelvic floor muscles, which meant that each day we had a few moments to see each other and to relax together. It played such an important role in our lives; soon

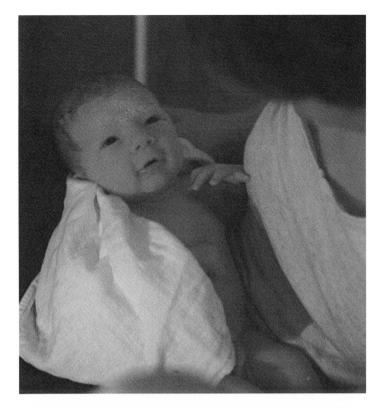

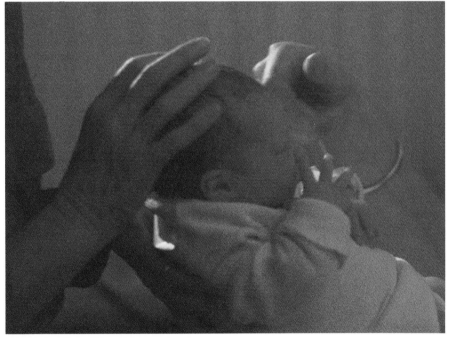

What was it like for you Rieke?

RIEKE: The whole event made a big impression on me. I was surprised by the beauty of the birth and the sight of such a lovely, tiny child. It made me want to have a child myself. The smooth course of the delivery and Dominique's tininess encouraged me. It is so wonderful to see a child coming out all bloody and watch how quickly it turns into a lovely baby.

GEERT: I was strongly affected by it as well. I had been able to discuss it abstractly, but, try as I might, I could never really picture it. I had tears in my eyes and was at a loss as to what to do. I walked around with her for a few moments, because I simply had to hold her. Not for long though because I was so excited. I practically started calling people, spreading the news. I knew that this was the most beautiful experience I had ever had. It took quite a while before I was able to talk about it calmly and not pour out a flood of feelings.

Did you have the help of a maternity nurse afterwards, or did you run everything by yourselves?

BETTINA: A maternity nurse came by once or twice a day. The rest of the time, Geert, Rieke, and my girlfriend Josje took care of me beautifully. They worked in shifts so someone was here day and night. I had ten days of marvelous pampering, during which I didn't have to lift a finger. That was fabulous. It was lovely to be surrounded all the time by people I love.

Josje, who has had some experience working as a maternity nurse, was here

we could have fun—go out, drink coffee somewhere, walk and bicycle together again—as we had done before the tensions arose.

What was first contact with Dominique like?

BETTINA: My body had worked so hard that I was almost unaware I had produced a baby. I kept thinking, 'My work is done, I want to rest, and I will attend to the child later.' She did not mean much to me then. The delivery was over, which had been an enormous job, and I didn't have much energy left. It took a few days before I liked her and enjoyed having her close to me. I was relieved that other people looked after her and cuddled her those first few days. I breastfed her and held her, but I felt the bonding would come in time, and it did.

for ten full days. Gerard and Rieke were going to take over when she went home, but things worked out quite differently. Even during the time that Josje was here, you two had your hands full.

When did you feel like taking over from them?

BETTINA: On the last day, Josje was here, so it worked out perfectly. I felt I was ready to be alone again and be with my baby without having the constant advice of others. The transition was very harmonious. At first, someone helped me with my laundry. Geert popped by every day and offered to do my shopping. This eased the transition from being taken care of totally to becoming independent again. The atmosphere at home was so good that I never felt hurried or pressured in any way. I could do everything at my own pace, surrendering to my rhythm and to what was happening inside me. I could simply take things as they came.

At first, you fed Dominique on demand. Has a regular rhythm been established?

BETTINA: A rhythm of sorts. She sleeps longer at night now. It took me a week to wean her off night feeds; they were too tiring for me. She is still a bit irregular in the daytime.

RIEKE: Her moods have a certain regularity, so I am getting to know her.

BETTINA: I was incredibly insecure during the first few weeks. 'What does she want, what shall I do, must I stick to a schedule and wake her up?' These questions burdened me. I expected she would clearly indicate everything he wanted, like falling asleep automatically when tired, or asking to be fed when hungry. Apparently, she had such an urge to suck that, were I to give into it, she would always be at my breast. So I had to regulate nursing to prevent her from snacking all day long. I try to feed her just six times a day, but she decides whether she drinks for one minute or for half an hour. I do not follow the suggested twenty-minute feedings.

GEERT: I can understand now what she means when she cries. I can hear whether she is tired or hungry. It is a different sound. Sometimes she whines and at other times she cries much more convincingly. Only a few things can be bothering her: a dirty diaper, hunger, or a burp.

How do you feel about your relationship with this child?

RIEKE: I love the sensation of holding the baby—feeling her body and giving her warmth and comfort. I do not feel in-hibited in any way. In adult relationships, there is always so much uncertainty before you touch someone or sit close to someone.

BETTINA: The intensity of the physical experience surprised me, too. The other day, Rieke and Dominique sat in the bath together. I enjoyed that a lot. I found it so nice to see how she moved around in the tub. I was totally elated by it, though, actually, nothing so special really happened. But there was something intense about it, from which I got great pleasure.

GEERT: It is a whole other world, which still somehow relates to the adult world. You learn something from it, and become sensitive to other people's feelings. Because babies can't say anything, you have to feel or see what they want. Still, I find it a pity they can't talk. This is the first baby that I've really liked. On one hand, I really quite enjoy this stage. On the other hand, I am looking forward to the time that she can come into my room to tell me stories.

BETTINA: You always think far ahead.

RIEKE: I'm just waiting for a smile. Now, the security and warmth I give her makes her quiet. When there is a sign of recognition, that will be enough for me.

ADJE AND REMY

Adje: Raoul's mother
Raoul: second child, a boy (born in hospital)
Gilles: first child, a boy (born at home)
Remy: Raoul's father

THE PHOTOGRAPHS IN THIS INTERVIEW WERE TAKEN WHEN RAOUL WAS THREE WEEKS OLD. ALREADY, AFTER HIS FEEDINGS, HE HAS INTENSE CHATS WITH ADJE. HE ORIENTS HIMSELF TO HER FACE AND VOICE AND TELLS HER, THROUGH A SURPRISING NUMBER OF FACIAL EXPRESSIONS, HOW HE EXPERIENCES HIS CONTACT WITH HER.

Is the first contact after the birth more intense than the contact which follows?

ADJE: Even now, I sometimes feel as if I experience the birth all over again. It may be at an odd moment in the middle of the day, or when I am all alone, or when my child looks at me suddenly and I look back and am moved. The first contact is very important, but when I have these moments now I think, 'Who is this new little person in my life?' It seems he wonders who I am, too.

What was that first contact, the moment your child was put on your belly, like?

ADJE: Fantastic. Very sensuous; he was very slippery and yet also firm. I knew I could direct all my emotions toward him, that I could surrender to him without inhibitions. I felt I could let him know who I was.

REMY: I certainly felt that way, too. My first reaction was to touch Raoul. He felt like a wet peach. The child's beauty evoked a deep emotional reaction; I felt strongly drawn to him. His coloring put me off a little bit—at first he reminded me of a hare. Babies look like game when they come out.

Do you feel he reacted to the way you held him and to your voice?

ADJE: Yes, very much so. I recall him searching, raising his head from time to time, touching, and caressing as an adult does.

REMY: It struck me that babies cry immediately after they are born. This doesn't last long. After they have contact with the mother, they become quiet and then crow with bliss. I find this marvelous. The moment they are taken away to be cleaned and dressed, they burst into tears again.

Did you know how to hold your first baby?

ADJE: It came naturally. And with Raoul, I never gave a minute's thought to how I should hold him. When I used to hold other people's babies now and then, it wasn't as easy. When I babysat I was always relieved when the mother left. The baby wasn't at ease as long as its mother was still around, whereas the child was fine when we were alone and we could get used to each other.

REMY: I was the first person to change his diaper, and I managed fine. But I feel a tremendous amount of concern for my child. When he is lying in his cradle and I've closed the door behind me, I think, 'I hope he isn't dead when I come back.'

ADJE: Gilles was born at eight o'clock on a still Sunday morning. No one else was around—no maternity nurse, no other family—just the three of us. Sitting with Remy in our big bed with Gilles in his cradle on the floor next to us was so

strange. I didn't feel at home with the new situation.

REMY: With Gilles, I didn't call the family for hours. With Raoul, I did this much sooner; I was so full with what had happened. The funny thing was that in the hospital I felt superfluous because they were doing things to both you and the baby. I didn't know whether to be with you or Raoul, so I paced from one of you to the other.

ADJE: I regret that I was less intimate with you during Raoul's birth. A nice attendant sat on my bed and calmed me down. You were out of it.

REMY: But I felt that I functioned much better this time because I was more down to earth about it. At Gilles' birth, I was rather frightened and emotional.

ADJE: I thought you were marvelous the first time. You did everything; I could concentrate totally on you. Everything else simply ceased to exist. This time, everything else dominated, which was a great pity. I never want to deliver in a hospital again, but I was intimidated because of my medical condition. I wouldn't do it again unless they came up with some very strong arguments for it.

How did Gilles take Raoul's arrival?

ADJE: In the beginning, everything went very easily, too easily really. He approved of everything.

REMY: Strangely, Gilles was the one who organized everybody in the days after his brother's birth. He let in visitors. On the staircase he would say, 'Be careful, don't fall,' and 'What would you like to drink?'

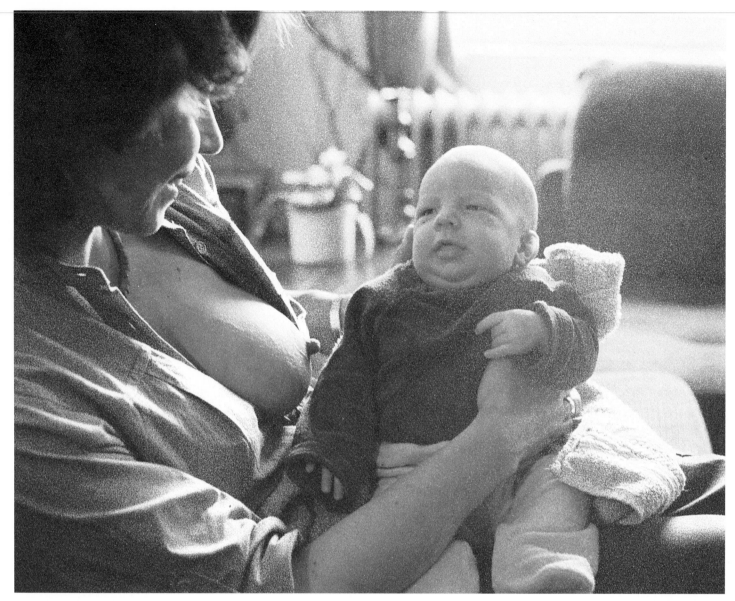

He was such the master of ceremonies that he was the center of attention.

ADJE: Looking back, I am glad it went so well with Gilles because I went through an unstable period. All kinds of questions and uncertainties hit me. He was very strong during this time. When I started to feel better, Gilles got depressed and emotional.

During the weeks after giving birth, did you dream more intensely and did you have stronger emotions than normal?

ADJE: I always dream anyway, but I was more emotional. Normally, you are part of society, but when you've delivered a baby you feel excluded from it. On the one hand, this is quite pleasant; on the other, I really long to be part of it again and to play a role. These feelings stayed with me for a long time after Gilles was born. Not so after Raoul—you have got to go on because another child depends on you. With Gilles I often felt lonely and rotten for no reason. I simply lost courage now and then.

I often wonder what the birth of a child is like for fathers. Remy, did you have some sort of emotional reaction?

REMY: That is hard to say because the period that follows the birth is so exhausting. You can't sleep normally. You wake up every few hours because the child has to be fed again. The first six to seven weeks were a true war of attrition.

ADJE: Remy used to get up and bring me the baby because I was too tired. With Gilles, my body took a long time to fully recover, even though I am rather strong physically. So much came at me. I was preoccupied with feeding. I felt that I pushed Remy into a corner with things like making love. After Gilles, it took three months before we could make love in a relaxed way again.

REMY: It isn't pleasant to make love immediately. You know that there are those stitches. You don't feel like it, you don't need it.

ADJE: As a woman, you still have the feeling of satisfaction because the child's sucking is sensual. You rarely feel like initiating sex with your partner.

REMY: You did during pregnancy. A pregnant woman with big breasts is delicious.

ADJE: Being pregnant is very liberating. You feel proud with your child inside you, and the three of you in bed is so cozy!

You breastfeed Raoul on demand, not according to set times. Does it take long before a certain rhythm is established?

ADJE: With both children, it took about six weeks. The moment the baby starts crying your body reacts with the letdown reflex. You can give your baby so much while you breastfeed. When Raoul is sad or something, the intimacy, if not the feeding itself, comforts him. After ten months, I had almost no milk left, but the moment I suckled Gilles I had a tie with him. For me, this period lasts about as long as the pregnancy: nine months pregnant, nine months feeding. Breastfeeding calms you down because you do nothing else while feeding. I get rather addicted to it.

You sometimes hear people say that a baby doesn't do much in those first few weeks after the birth except eat and sleep. What was your experience?

ADJE: The baby and I were both recovering. We had moments during those weeks when we would temporarily wake up from a long, deep sleep. After about ten days, you both start to wake up, play, respond to each other, and have fun doing so. The tiny baby can concentrate already for a few minutes. I think a baby responds from the very beginning: being elated, sad, tired. He and I were one. There was complete harmony.

With a baby, you have a different sort of communication than with adults, with whom you use language, words, which you say now seems a roundabout way of communicating.

ADJE: When you have a relationship with an adult, you develop a specific way of interacting with each other even though you never plan it. It is different with a baby. There is nothing to hide, no holding back. I think that is fantastic.

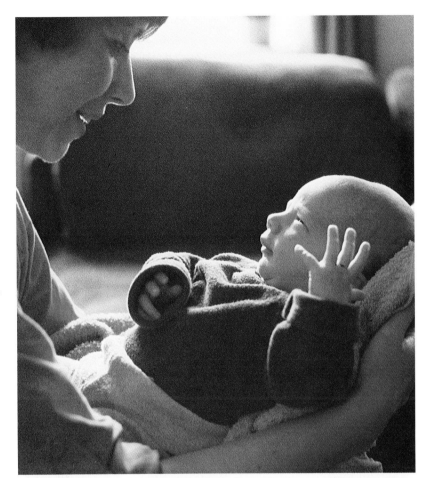

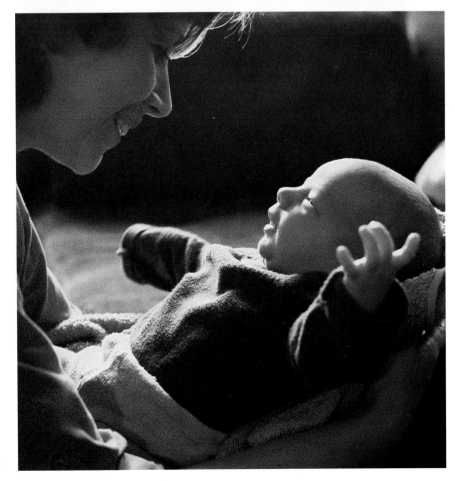

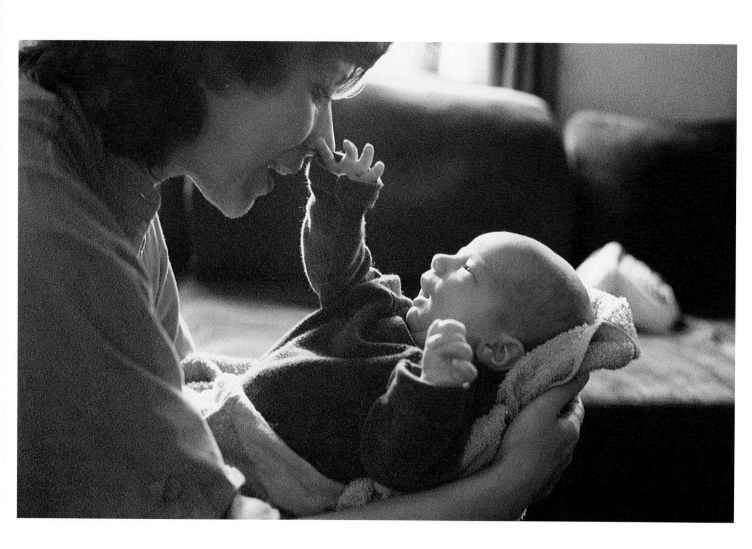

JEROEN

Jeroen: Veertje's father
Veertje: first child, a girl (born in hospital)
Elke: Veertje's mother
Johan: gynecologist

THIS INTERVIEW TOOK PLACE FOUR WEEKS AFTER VEERTJE'S BIRTH. THE PHOTOGRAPHS WERE TAKEN AT THAT TIME.

The birth of a child is a very emotional occasion for the mother. What is it like for the father?

JEROEN: It was a sort of meditation. Waiting for what was happening, a natural process, which lasts for hours.

Did you feel that you would like to do something, rather than just wait?

Elke asked me to massage her lower back. I massaged when a contraction started. That was not 'doing.' That was a treatment repeated one hundred times or more, a sort of ritual. Elke was absent then, she drew into herself, and had no actual contact with me. I think that is why I got the feeling of meditating—you don't really communicate with each other, but together undergo the natural process of the contractions coming and going.

Was this Elke's experience also?

I've asked her how she experienced my presence. She described it as extremely calming. She did not realize that I felt like I was nearly in a trance. The whole birth process lasted from about ten o'clock until six. It intensifies as it progresses.

From what position did Elke push?

A position that neither of us had thought of in advance. Elke wanted to deal with the contractions on her hands and knees while rocking. I squatted in front of her. She found it pleasant to rock with her head up against me or in my lap.

She raised herself up to push. She also sat up straight, threw her arms round my neck, and pushed. She pulled very hard on my neck. I had to brace myself. Michel Odent says the delivering woman needs a force to oppose the forces that pull her downward.

Did you feel at one with Elke during the pushing? Did you feel that you were inwardly pushing, too?

No, I did not feel that I was sharing what Elke was feeling. I merely observed and that was very moving. It was much more of a complementary relationship. She needed to hug me, to pull on me, and to lie in my lap. That fitted exactly with my needs. It is wonderful to have birth take place very close to you, to feel, see, and smell. Actually, as a continuation of a loving experience. I think it was so for her, too; yet, afterwards, she had the impression that she was overwhelmed by pain.

Did you find her pain unpleasant?

I felt that she regressed. That she was struggling to control herself but eventually could not succeed. She became like a very small child who was afraid of the pain and sought shelter and protection. The fear of the pain was closely linked to the feeling that she was no longer in control and did not know what was happening and where it would all end.

Was it warm in the hospital?

I did not find it warm enough. We had a small room in which the heat was turned way up, but it was not warm enough for me. In order to get warmer, we crept under a thick blanket.

How were the first moments after Veertje's birth?

She was given to Elke who could not lift her up because the cord was too short. Also, Elke was tired and got the shivers from exerting herself. You can't make a good first contact with the baby when you're weak. When Johan, the gynecologist, was dealing with Veertje, I paid more attention to the cord than to the baby. I saw the cord pulsating powerfully and knew that the baby was being soundly fed. The baby's cord was cut, and she was dressed by the nurse which was a good thing because it was not so warm. Johan took her again for a bit to look her over. It occurred to me that Veertje was terribly disturbed by all the handling. I did not find her beautiful when I saw her like that. She looked ugly and unhappy. Then she was put in the cradle that was heated by hot-water bottles.

You still had not held her?

No. They were very involved in medical procedures. First, they tucked in the baby and then dealt with Elke. She had torn and needed to be stitched. The cradle was nearby. I took Veertje out of the cradle, actually with the intention of giving her back to Elke. I thought it might help stop the shivers. I found it awful that she shivered so much that her teeth chattered. As I picked up Veertje she opened her eyes very wide and immediately searched for my face. She did not cry, and I started

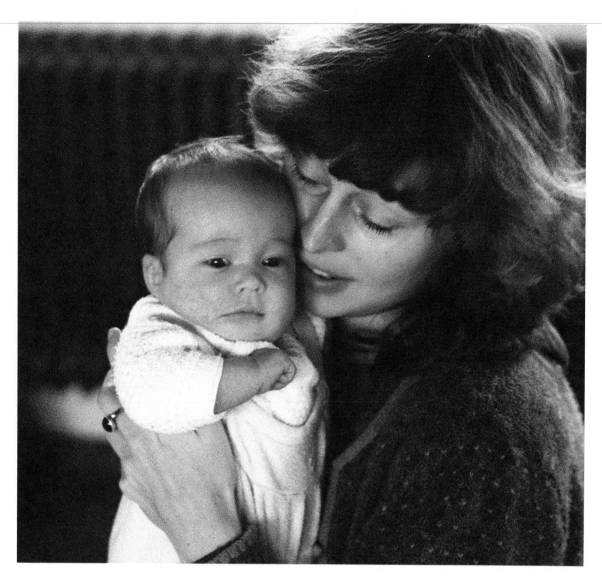

to talk to her spontaneously. She sought very hard for eye contact, looked through me almost, and began to smile. She was very happy.

I was extremely surprised because I was sure that I, too, would be a set of strange hands to her. I had the idea that only the mother's movements are trusted by a newborn child. I thought, 'she looks at me as though she knows me, and she clearly trusts me to carry her.' I realized later that the baby was already responding to our voices before the birth. During the last months of pregnancy, the baby listens intently to the noises in the house and follows the voices of the mother and father and other people it hears frequently and responds by moving. I saw that she recognized me. This moment was a continuation of the happiness I felt during the

birth. That wonderful searching of hers, that relaxed little face, that smile. She continued to make faces for a couple of days afterwards.

Elke was shivering for quite some time, about ten minutes. Then, she was involved with the afterbirth and the stitching. Veertje felt just fine with me. I could not let her go. I was talking to her and was captivated by her way of looking at me from close up. Really looking in the eyes, much more capably than I had expected, and answering with her fine lips, which didn't have the hard marks on them from sucking yet. I had the feeling that she was responding to what I was telling her by using her puckered little lips.

Her answer was silent?
Yes, she just made all sorts of faces.

Naturally, she sometimes looked away. You could see that she was listening intently. She did this consistently when she heard Elke's voice. Elke's voice made her very inquisitive. She started to look and listen; she got a pretty little expression. At a certain moment, Elke felt well enough to take the child to her breast. I believe Elke reacted to the way Veertje moved her mouth, from which you could see that she wanted to nurse. She fed very briefly but long enough for the midwife to ensure that the sucking reflex was working well. I had expected her to drink more diligently and not give up so quickly. She drank for a bit and then started to look round again; she was extremely busy looking. After a good hour, she fell asleep. An hour or two later, she woke up and resumed the intensive contact. I had ex-

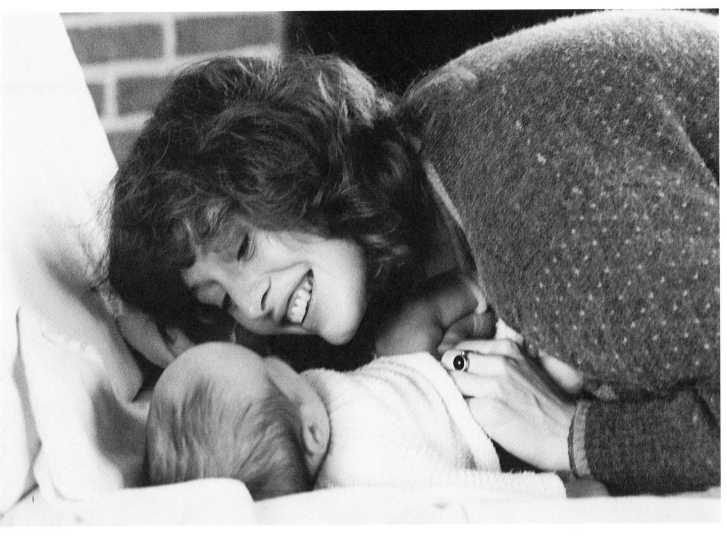

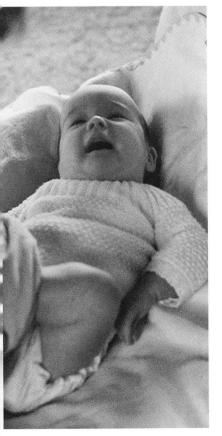

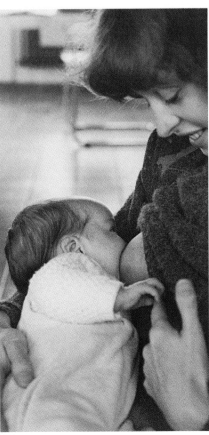

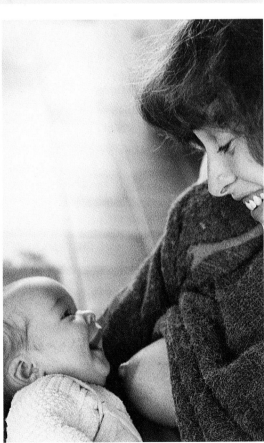

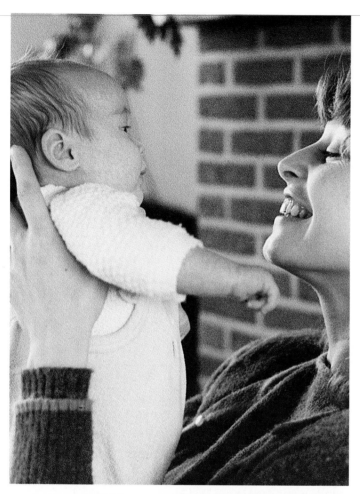
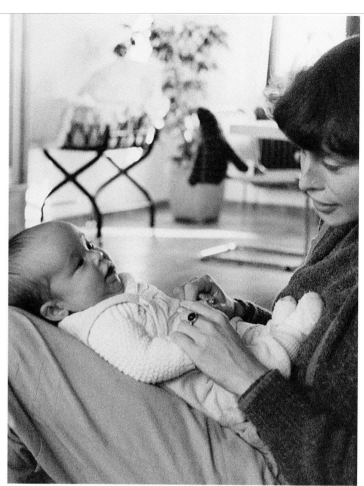
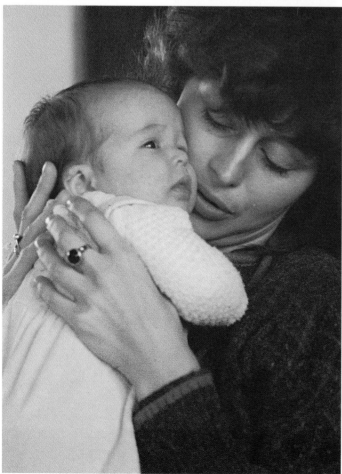
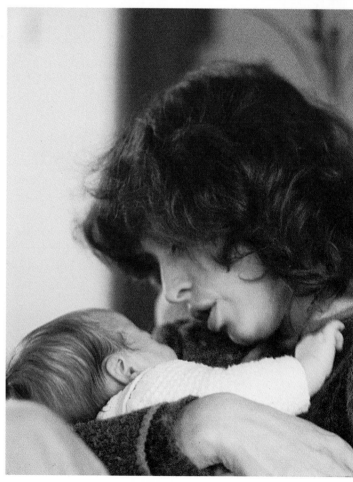

pected the baby would be very awake at first contact as a result of the stress of the birth and then take several days to recover. She did not do that. She slept and then had energy for yet more exploration; she looked and laughed. As soon as she woke up she wanted contact.

She was very involved with you two. How was it at night? Where did she sleep?

In the day, she had no problem being in the cradle downstairs. It was warm there. She could hear familiar sounds. At night, lying in her cot by our bed, she would wake up after half an hour and cry. We'd move her into bed with us and then everything was okay. This continued for the first week and a half. Suddenly, it was not necessary anymore. At one stage, she could sleep in the cradle at night, and if she woke up, could, without panicking, make noises to tell us that she wanted contact and wanted to eat.

Does she use her voice quite a bit?

Veertje produced sounds from her throat very soon after she was born. A variety of grunts emerged. She would make sounds upon waking, during stretching, or when she simply felt comfortable. She shared her experiences in this way. In the first few weeks, these sounds were musical, very soft, and very spontaneous with lots of variation. From the second week on, her sounds became more specific. They clearly expressed displeasure, pleasure, or sleepiness. She makes fewer sounds now, but they are much clearer and also somewhat louder than before.

Has she become more confident?

She has much more self-confidence. For ten days or so, Veertje was not able to control her hands and head. From the

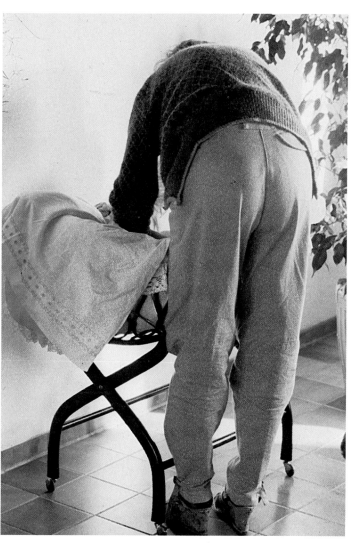

first days on, she concentrated on finding her hands and looking at them. When she succeeded at getting her hands into her field of vision, she would try to achieve it again and would put her hands into her mouth or against her cheeks. She was grateful when I assisted her. I got into the habit of moving her hand to her mouth when she made sucking motions or when she wasn't feeling well. She seemed to enjoy sucking her hand.

Earlier than I had expected, in the second week, she watched her hands while lying on her side in the cradle and then deliberately brought them to her mouth. Now, she can bring both hands together, hold hands, cross her fingers, and play with her hands. She sucks her hands but also uses them to explore her face. I feel this reassures her and makes her happy.

Did you enjoy looking after the baby?

A week after her birth, I got the flu, and the doctor told me not to touch the baby until the danger of giving it to her passed. From the moment I could no longer carry or touch the baby, I had negative feelings toward her. It made me think about child abuse. People who do that must have negative feelings about the baby's behavior or inaccessibility. If I was alone in the room with the baby and she cried because she had heard Elke go out, I had great difficulty pacifying her. I could not cuddle or stroke her. I'd think 'shut your boring mouth.' I began to have doubts about myself. I had the idea that I hated my child.

I thought that if I couldn't stroke, I would hit. I became very conscious of the reasons for child abuse, of incubator babies in particular. If you can't stroke, there is a gap in the communication between the baby and its parents. The baby doesn't expect you to keep your distance. She looks for you, sees you, and expects you to stroke her, pick her up, and cuddle her. If that does not happen, the baby looks at you worriedly. Distance is alienating. The baby then behaves badly—whines, cries, and jerks. That made me feel dislike for Veertje. Nevertheless, I was stuck with the order not to cuddle her.

How long did it take for your feelings of dislike to pass?

I started to cuddle her again after ten days, and all my feelings of alienation and irritation toward her, as well as her fear of me because I had kept my distance, went away at once. Everything was good. I could identify again with what the baby was feeling and with what was going on between her and Elke.

You have said that the first contact with your

child is unbelievably open and intense and that intensity never comes back.

After four weeks experience I still feel that way. Although, I certainly was surprised in those first days after the birth that she continued to seek such direct eye contact and to give signs of recognition, a sort of greeting. The length of time she did this was much shorter than during the first contact; being engrossed with each other for an hour stretch has not come back. What does happen now is in the morning as it gets light she behaves almost as she did at the first contact. Immediately after feeding, she is very interested in looking around; she smiles and expresses herself. That is not so apparent during the rest of the day. In the morning—and I had this feeling in the first contact also—you get a clear answer to the contact you make.

At other times of day, she does not give any answer if I seek contact but forces me to wait until she makes contact. She likes it a lot when I hold her, creating an intimate atmosphere, but I must not be too active. I seem to have difficulty with that; I don't always have the patience or the time to wait until the baby deigns to look at me. But when I relax and am with her for a bit, she responds. I believe she can hear from my breathing if I am really relaxed.

Another thing I had not appreciated initially was that the baby can move her head up and down as well as left and right. I don't know if this is because she was a breech delivery, but immediately after the birth, she pulled her head in deep between her shoulders. Her neck got longer every day. She still pulls her head in completely and then sticks it out. If the back of her head is well supported, she can stick her head out far and look at you particularly alertly. If you don't support the head, she is preoccupied with balance and has little energy left for being inquisitive. Support of the head is an invitation to make contact. If she accepts, she sticks up her head; if she rejects you, she pulls back her chin.

As soon as she gets hungry, she looks at me disapprovingly. I am the father. She knows I have nothing for her and wants to go to her mother. I am to have contact with the baby only when she feels good, not when she is hungry or sleepy. At those times, she has to be with Elke. She makes this very obvious.

A baby has changing interests. You must not do the same thing over and over because that gets dull, but you also can't introduce too much at one time that is new because the baby may find this frightening. When she was very young, Veertje found it delightful to be held in front of the window. To please her, I put her by the window in a fruit basket. For a couple of days, she preferred this to anything else. It looked sweet—a week-old baby on the windowsill enjoying the light pouring in. Then her fascination with that disappeared.

What I can see in her eyes has made a great impression on me. I really see the intensity with which she receives me. The way she looks at me gives me a feeling of nudity. In the second week, Veertje was extremely involved in the world of noises, listening very intensively, particularly to all new sounds. By chance, there were storms during that time. She could not sleep; she was listening to the rain and the wind. She strained to listen, her eyes open but unseeing; she got upset if I tried to make eye contact, as if she was thinking 'Get out of my way; I am listening.'

Suggested Reading

PREGNANCY AND CHILDBIRTH

Armstrong, Penny and Sheryl Feldman: *Wise Birth: Bringing Together the Best of Natural Childbirth with Modern Medicine* (New York: Quill, 1991). How to find a setting that will make birth a healthy and positive experience.

Balaskas, Janet: *Active Birth: The New Approach to Giving Birth Naturally.* rev. ed., ed. Linda Ziedrich (Boston: Harvard Common Press, 1992). A guide to movement in pregnancy, birth, and the postnatal period. Helps women develop their physical resources for labor and birth.

Balaskas, Janet: *Natural Pregnancy* (Brooklyn, NY: Interlink Publishing Group, 1990). A practical, holistic guide to well-being from conception to birth through diet, exercise, yoga, massage, and holistic healing.

Balaskas, Janet: *Water Birth: The Concise Guide to Using Water During Pregnancy, Birth, and Infancy* (San Francisco: Thorsons, 1992). How water can be used during pregnancy and childbirth, also includes baby massage and teaching babies to swim.

Baldwin, Rahima and Terra Palmarini: *Pregnant Feelings.* rev. ed. (Berkeley, CA: Celestial Arts, 1986). Practical self-help approach to the emotional facet of birth.

Baldwin, Rahima: *Special Delivery* (Berkeley, CA: Celestial Arts, 1986). Practical guide for couples who want greater responsibility for the birth of their babies, with sections on hospital options, Cesarean prevention, and emotional aspects of birth.

Chalmers, Iain, Murray Enkin and Marc Keirse, eds.: *Effective Care in Pregnancy and Childbirth.* 2 vols. (New York: Oxford University Press, 1989). A comprehensive, systematic review of the effects of care during pregnancy and childbirth, based on over 3,000 clinical research studies from 1950 to date.

Enkin, Keirse and Chalmers: *Guide to Effective Care in Pregnancy and Childbirth* (New York: Oxford University Press, 1989). The main findings and conclusions of Chalmers, but without references.

Goldsmith, Judith: *Childbirth Wisdom: From the World's Oldest Societies* (Brookline, MA: East West Health Books, 1990). Information about traditional birth practices that sheds new light on contemporary practices.

Jordan, Sandra: *Yoga for Pregnancy: Ninety-Two Safe, Gentle Stretches Appropriate for Pregnant Women and New Mothers* (New York: St. Martin's Press, 1988). Ninety-two Iyengar poses chosen for safety and effectiveness in pregnancy.

Kitzinger, Sheila: *Complete Book of Pregnancy and Childbirth.* rev. and exp. (New York: Knopf, 1989). Comprehensive, splendidly illustrated reference guide by the international expert.

Kitzinger, Sheila: *Homebirth* (New York: Dorling Kindersley, 1991). A commonsense guide for women considering alternatives to giving birth in the hospital.

Kitzinger, Sheila, ed.: *Midwife Challenge.* rev. ed. (San Francisco: Pandora Press, 1991). Compares the situation of midwives in different countries, the problems they face, their hopes for the future.

Leboyer, Frederick: *Birth Without Violence* (New York: Fawcett Book Group, 1990). Poetic and powerful plea to make birth more peaceful for the vulnerable, sensitive newborn.

Lim, Robin: *After the Baby's Birth: A Woman's Way to Wellness* (Berkeley, CA: Celestial Arts, 1991). Helps women and their families learn how to have a healthier, saner postpartum experience.

Nilsson, Lennert: *A Child Is Born* (New York: Delecorte Press, 1990). Human reproduction—conception to birth—with outstanding photographs.

Newton, Niles: *Newton on Birth and Women: Selected Works of Niles Newton, Both Classic and Current* (Seattle: Birth and Life Bookstore, 1990). Classic and important articles and speeches by Niles Newton and associates.

Odent, Michel: *Birth Reborn* (New York: Pantheon Books, 1986). Description of birth at Pithiviers, France. Shows how birth can be a natural and safe part of life and how a woman can approach delivery with confidence.

Odent, Michel: *Water and Sexuality* (New York: Penguin Books, 1990). A vision of humans as aquatic primates, explored through water birth and eroticism, as well as in myth, legend, metaphor, and even advertising.

Olkin, Sylvia Klein: *Positive Pregnancy Fitness: A Guide to a More Comfortable Pregnancy and Easier Birth Through Exercise and Relaxation* (Garden City Park, NY: Avery Publishing Group, 1987). Mental, physical, and spiritual preparation for pregnancy and birth, using yoga, exercise, and relaxation.

Rothman, Barbara Katz: *In Labor: Women and Power in the Birthplace* (New York: W. W. Norton, 1991). Analyzes not only how childbirth is managed in America but why it is managed this way.

Rothman, Barbara Katz: *Recreating Motherhood: Ideology and Technology in a Patriarchal Society* (New York: W. W. Norton, 1989). Examines how the real needs of mother, father, and child have been swept aside in an attempt to reduce the complex and wondrous process of birth to a clinical event that can be controlled by medical technology.

Sidenbladh, Erik: *Water Babies: The Igor Tjarkovsky Method for Delivery in Water,* trans. Wendy Croton (New York: St. Martin's Press, 1983). The theories of Igor Tjarkovsky on underwater childbirth and infant swimming.

Simkin, Penny: *Birth Partner: Everything You Need to Know to Help a Woman Through Childbirth* (Boston: Harvard Common Press, 1989). An outstanding childbirth educator offers a complete and practical guide to help ensure that birth is fulfilling for the mother.

Simkin, Penny, Janet Whalley and Ann Keppler: *Pregnancy, Childbirth, and the Newborn.* rev. ed. (Deerhaven, MN: Meadowbrook Press, 1991). Information to assist parents in developing their own ways of giving birth. Reflects the latest changes in obstetric technology and offers new coping strategies.

Wertz, Richard W. and Dorothy C. Wertz: *Lying-in: A History of Childbirth in America* (New Haven, CT: Yale University Press, 1989). Looks at the effects of hospitals on deliveries in the United States from colonial times to the present.

BREASTFEEDING

Huggins, Kathleen: *Nursing Mother's Companion.* rev. ed. (Boston: Harvard Common Press, 1991). A lucid, trouble-shooting aid for the new mother as she learns how to nurse.

Kitzinger, Sheila: *Breastfeeding Your Baby* (New York: Knopf, 1989). Reassuring breast-feeding guide, with outstanding photos and illustrations, many in color.

Palmer, Gabrielle: *Politics of Breastfeeding* (New York: Unwin Hyman, 1989). A cross-cultural study of political and social pressures toward artificial feeding.

Renfrew, Mary, Chloe Fisher and Suzanne Arms: *Bestfeeding* (Berkeley, CA: Celestial Arts, 1990). A clear, basic breastfeeding guide—how to get started and how to solve problems, with accurate information and pictures.

VIDEOS

Netherlands Association of Midwives: *Home Birth in Holland,* 45 min. 1990. (Highlight Productions) Prenatal care, three home births, and postnatal care attended by midwives, emphasizes normalcy of birth.

St. Charles, Elize: *Modern Moves for Pregnancy Fitness,* 60 min. 1990. (St. Charles and Associates) Conditioning and stress reduction program combines yoga stretches with contemporary nonimpact exercise for women before and after childbirth.

These books and videos are available at your local bookstore or from Birth and Life Bookstore, P.O. Box 70625, Seattle, Washington 98107 (toll-free phone United States and Canada: (800) 736-0631).

INDEX

More books on women's health and family issues...

HEART & HANDS by Elizabeth Davis

This comprehensive and classic "midwife's guide" to pregnancy and birth demystifies modern obstetrics and provides sound guidelines for alternative care. Illustrated with line drawings and more than 60 photographs by Suzanne Arms. Revised and updated. *$19.95 paper or $22.95 cloth, 248 pages*

AFTER THE BABY'S BIRTH . . . A WOMAN'S WAY TO WELLNESS
by Robin Lim

This complete guide to postpartum care for mother and baby focuses on natural and wholesome practices. Illustrated throughout, this warm, sensitive text has advice on parental nurturing, breastfeeding, nutrition, pelvic health, early education, the role of the father, and the all-importance of love. *$14.95 paper, 272 pages*

BESTFEEDING: GETTING BREASTFEEDING RIGHT FOR YOU
by Mary Renfrew, Chloe Fisher, and Suzanne Arms

Midwives have known for years that women who breastfeed have healthier, happier children, but few new mothers anticipate problems or realize that breastfeeding is rarely easy or instinctive. This complete and practical guidebook, filled with photos and illustrations, gives mothers support and detailed advice for dealing with common situations. *$12.95 paper, 240 pages*

THE INFERTILITY BOOK by Carla Harkness

With the experience of ten years testing and treatment, the author expertly and sensitively discusses the emotional, physical, and social effects of infertility. The book also details the latest medical breakthroughs and procedures. Created with the help of specialists, psychologists, counselors, fellow patients, surrogate mothers, and biological and adoptive parents, this is the sourcebook for anyone facing one of the most heartbreaking and mysterious problems of our times. *$14.95 paper, 360 pages*

IMMACULATE DECEPTION: BIRTH AND BEYOND by Suzanne Arms

Over fifteen years ago, Suzanne Arms revolutionized the way we think about giving birth with *Immaculate Deception: A New Look at Women and Childbirth*. Part exposé, part prescription for change, this book broke the silence surrounding intrusive and sometimes deadly birthing methods and suggested a safer and more natural way. Fully revised and updated, *Immaculate Deception: Birth and Beyond* has new interviews, photos, and the latest medical data incorporated with traditional wisdom. *$14.95 paper, 284 pages*

SPECIAL DELIVERY by Rahima Baldwin

Midwife, childbirth educator, and internationally-known speaker Rahima Baldwin presents a guide to structuring the birth experience you want for yourself and your baby. Chapters cover choosing hospital or home birth, prenatal care, handling labor, dealing with complications, and more. *$14.95 paper, 192 pages*

PREGNANT FEELINGS
by Rahima Baldwin & Terra Palmarini Richardson

This workbook for pregnant women and their partners helps them to recognize and work with the emotions and energies surrounding pregnancy and birth. Practical exercises lead to a sense of self-confidence and power in new and not-so-new parents. *$14.95 paper, 208 pages*

ENERGETIC PREGNANCY by Elizabeth Davis

"...a wonderful gift of a book...Davis's great knowledge of women's health and her long experience working with childbearing women combine well with her intuition and gentle approach to personal growth."—*The Birth Gazette*
A guide to health and vitality from conception through birth and beyond. *$8.95 paper, 172 pages*

YOU ARE YOUR CHILD'S FIRST TEACHER by Rahima Baldwin

An exciting new vision of parenting in which parents have an active educational role from the moment of birth. Drawing on child development research, Baldwin details how to nurture your child's mind, body, emotions, and imagination. *$12.95 paper or $19.95 cloth, 380 pages*

Available from your local bookstore, or order direct from the publisher. Please include $2.50 shipping & handling for the first book, and 50¢ for each additional book. California residents include local sales tax. Write for our free complete catalog of over 400 books, posters, and tapes.

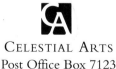

CELESTIAL ARTS
Post Office Box 7123
Berkeley, California 94707
For VISA or MasterCard orders, call (510) 845-8414